D1426893

SURGEON
AT WAR
1939–45

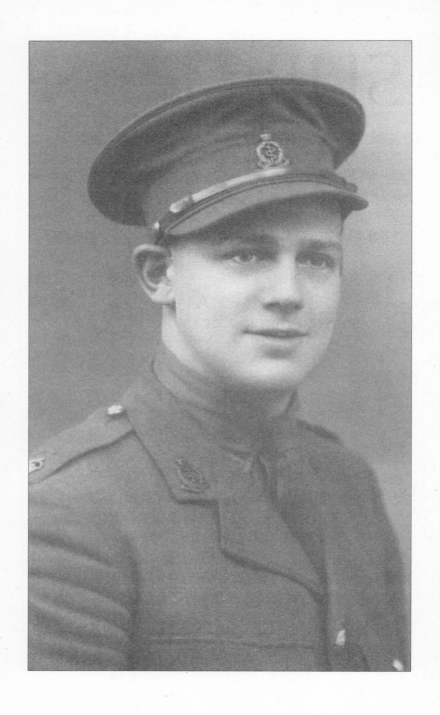

SURGEON
AT WAR
1939–45

THE SECOND WORLD WAR SEEN FROM OPERATING
TABLES BEHIND THE FRONT LINE

STANLEY AYLETT
EDITED AND INTRODUCED BY HOLLY AYLETT

metro

First published by Metro Publishing,
an imprint of
John Blake Publishing Limited
3 Bramber Court, 2 Bramber Road
London W14 9PB

www.johnblakepublishing.co.uk

www.facebook.com/johnblakebooks ⓕ
twitter.com/jblakebooks ⓔ

First published in hardback in 2015

ISBN: 978-1-78418-124-6

British Library Cataloguing-in-Publication Data:

A catalogue record for this book is available from the British Library.

Design by www.envydesign.co.uk

Printed in Great Britain by CPI Group (UK) Ltd

1 3 5 7 9 10 8 6 4 2

Papers used by John Blake Publishing are natural, recyclable products made
from wood grown in sustainable forests. The manufacturing processes conform
to the environmental regulations of the country of origin.

Every attempt has been made to contact the relevant copyright-holders,
but some were unobtainable. We would be grateful if the
appropriate people could contact us.

For my father's grandchildren, Christopher, Rose, Ralph, Aidan, and Anna-Clare.

The original, privately published, edition of this book was dedicated to the officers and other ranks of the Royal Army Medical Corps and to the nurses of the Queen Alexandra's Imperial Nursing Service with whom my father served.

I would like to acknowledge with special thanks the support given by Kay Aylett, and Antony and Rosemary Gray

CONTENTS

DEDICATION AND ACKNOWLEDGEMENTS   v

INTRODUCTION TO THE SECOND EDITION   xiii

AUTHOR'S PREFACE   xxi

1   THE DAYS PRECEDING THE OUTBREAK OF WAR   1
     SEPTEMBER–NOVEMBER 1939

2   SETTING UP HOSPITAL IN FRANCE   11
     The 'phoney war'; setting up No. 6 General Hospital outside
     Le Tréport; visit to Paris; a German agent befriended
     NOVEMBER 1939–MAY 1940

3   THE GERMAN BLITZKRIEG ON BELGIUM   29
     AND FRANCE
     In forward areas with No. 159 Welsh Field Ambulance near Ypres
     and elsewhere in Belgium; retreat through France to Dunkirk;
     rescue by HMS Havant *and return to Dover*
     MAY–JUNE 1940

4   CREATING A HOSPITAL AT DOVER   53
    From Leeds to Dover and a false alarm
    JUNE–SEPTEMBER 1940

5   ORGANISATION OF THE RAMC   63
    No. 6 General Hospital, Luton; to London for course on
    tropical diseases
    OCTOBER–NOVEMBER 1940

6   VOYAGE TO SUEZ   73
    Embarkation on Clydeside; voyage to Suez and life aboard
    the Nea Hellas *with stopover in Durban*
    NOVEMBER 1940–FEBRUARY 1941

7   LANDING AT SUEZ   91
    The vast encampment at El Quassasin; the first of many visits
    to Cairo
    FEBRUARY–MARCH 1941

8   A COURT MARTIAL AND SUBSEQUENT   103
    POSTING
    From the witness box in Cairo to duties at No. 64 General
    Hospital in Alexandria
    APRIL –MAY 1941

9   NON-MEDICAL DUTIES IN A GENERAL   123
    HOSPITAL
    Recreational activities; breaks in Alexandria; visit to the Holy Land
    JUNE 1941–FEBRUARY 1942

10 INCIDENTS AT THE HOSPITAL   137
    Congeniality of the workplace; eccentric colleagues, in particular
    Major Geoffrey Morley; visit to the Upper Nile
    JUNE 1941–FEBRUARY 1942

11 DEPARTURE FOR THE DESERT   157
    Attached to an Indian casualty clearing station along the
    coast before being posted to Tobruk
    MARCH–MAY 1942

12 THE MOVE TO TOBRUK   177
    Conditions in the Tobruk hospital; retreat with the Eighth Army;
    return to No. 64 General Hospital, Alexandria
    MAY–JUNE 1942

13 THE EXODUS FROM ALEXANDRIA   191
    In the desert before the battle of El Alamein; return to
    Alexandria; casualties at No. 64 General Hospital;
    victory and the arrival of spring
    JULY 1942–MAY 1943

14 WORK IN A PLASTIC UNIT AND NO. 10 CCS   209
    From Alexandria to a plastic-surgery unit in Cairo; No. 10
    Casualty Clearing Station outside Tobruk; return to Glasgow
    JUNE–DECEMBER 1943

15 CHRISTMAS AT HOME AND PREPARATIONS   227
    FOR D-DAY
    Family reunion in London; to Cambridge to prepare No. 10
    Casualty Clearing Station for D-Day; appointed to command
    No. 14 Field Surgical Unit
    DECEMBER 1943–JUNE 1944

16 D-DAY AND ITS AFTERMATH   249
    Normandy landings, 6 June 1944; CCS set up near Bayeux;
    dealing with casualties and an incompetent anaesthetist
    JUNE 1944

17 THE ADVANCE ACROSS FRANCE AND BELGIUM 269
    INTO HOLLAND
    Keeping up with the advance towards Paris; visit to liberated
    Paris; on into Belgium; visit to liberated Brussels; entry into
    Holland; attached to CCS at Nijmegen
    JULY–SEPTEMBER 1944

18 ENTRY INTO GERMANY   289
    On to Eisden then return to Nijmegen; posted to join a
    Canadian CCS in Germany; rejoining No. 10 CCS at Schloss
    Wissen; crossing of the Rhine
    SEPTEMBER 1944–MARCH 1945

19 UNCOVERING A CONCENTRATION CAMP   311
    On leave in Paris; return via Brussels to No. 3 CCS;
    rejoining No. 10 CCS near Bremen; VE-Day amid the
    horror of a concentration camp near Sandbostel; goodbye to
    No. 10 CCS
    APRIL–MAY 1945

20 CLEARING THE WOUNDED IN DENMARK   333
    To Copenhagen via Cuxhaven; assessing the German wounded
    in Zealand hospitals; usefulness of cigarettes; goodbye to
    No. 14 FSU and to Hanover via Flensburg
    JUNE–JULY 1945

EPILOGUE   349
  Final posting to hospital in Hanover; return to England;
  discharge at Albany Street Barracks; back on the wards at
  King's College Hospital
  JULY–OCTOBER 1945

AFTERWORD   357

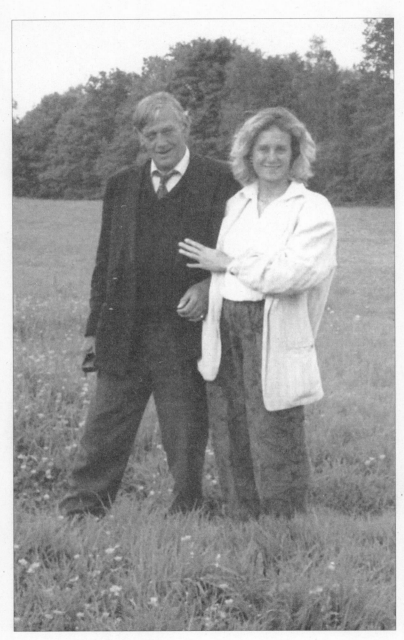

The author with his daughter, *circa* 1983.

INTRODUCTION TO THE SECOND EDITION

On the night before he died, I was sitting at my father's bedside when he said to me, 'I don't think I could have done more with my life.' It was the reckoning of a man who had reached the end and was trying to evaluate his story. There was something tentative in the statement, which begged the question: Could I have done more? The question was impossible to answer, but it spoke of a deep sense of moral imperative, which evolved in the young man we see ageing rapidly in the pages of this book and that remained a driving force throughout his life. He had resolved to dedicate his considerable skills to the service of medicine, and in the defence of life. But who could measure such a commitment? I felt his love in sharing this reflection with me. I also felt that coming from a different generation, and with over forty years between us, I could never be his judge.

My father wrote this memoir when he was nearing retirement in his late sixties. He was looking back at the man he was in 1939 when he signed up to join the Royal Army Medical Corps in the week after war was declared. He was twenty-eight. He had qualified at King's College in London with distinction, practised as a registrar and spent one year as a ship's surgeon on a merchant ship which sailed as far as the China Sea. At the time, King's College was not encouraging its staff to enlist, so he left with a sense of duty but without the college's blessing.

He spent the early part of the war setting up a large field hospital in Normandy, before moving to the front in May 1940. After the invasion of the Low Countries and France, his surgical unit retreated with their wounded to the beaches near Dunkirk. Here they joined the exodus and only narrowly survived the crossing, when they were rescued from their sinking boat, mid-Channel, by the destroyer HMS *Havant*. Then, after a short course in tropical medicine, he sailed to Egypt in January 1941 as part of the Middle East Force, serving both at the base hospital in Alexandria and behind the front lines in the desert. Over two and a half years later, in November 1943, he returned to England to take part in preparations for the invasion and was sent into France with the British Liberation Force the day after D-Day in June 1944. When VE-Day came, almost a year later, he and his unit were engaged in opening up the Sandbostel concentration camp, near Bremen in Germany. Finally, after some weeks clearing German prisoners of war from hospitals in Denmark, he returned to England and re-entered civilian life in October 1945.

It was an epic journey – over seven years and two continents. He lived through changes in the organisation of the Royal Army Medical Corps, in the drugs available (there was no penicillin at first) and the medical equipment. This was the last Western war where doctors would carry out major operations with post-operative wards close behind the front line. Initially, surgeons were organised in small units and dependent on the facilities of the casualty clearing stations to be able to operate. It was not until 1944 that the Royal Army Medical Corps perfected its field service units so that a surgeon with his anaesthetist could function autonomously with their own theatre, a twelve-bed ward, two three-ton lorries and a couple of orderlies.

In the midst of the worst carnage, surgeons would be operating for seventeen-hour stretches, followed by time in the wards, for days on end, making hundreds of quick decisions without the benefit of diagnostic aids. Then, three hours to pack up, a few hours' sleep, a journey through devastation, three hours in which to set up, and it would all start again.

In the early stages my father sometimes kept count — three hundred and five operations in fourteen days on one occasion. Later he just kept going. Surprisingly, he records few times when the teams were unable to keep up with the numbers of wounded. In this parallel battle behind the front line, surgeons were driven to take risks against all odds so long as there was the least chance of saving a soldier from death. Amid the sickening sight of youth being slaughtered, saving lives became a mission, and the compassion and engagement with each soldier at their most vulnerable moment was an affirmation of humanity in a landscape of destruction, heroism and depravity. Delivered to the safety of the other side, my father recalls how, back on the peacetime streets of London, he could still conjure up the faces of his patients, 'row upon row of them, with all the courage that masked their pain and made light of their suffering'.

Although he had chosen to spend these years in service, a decision he never regretted, this story is also one of a young man trying to prepare for his future. He was aware of the professional limitations of war surgery in comparison with civilian surgery, and sometimes missed engagement with a broader academic field of medicine. In moments of self-doubt he feared this might prevent him from realising his student ambition to become a leading consultant surgeon. Ironically, it proved the opposite. During the calmer months in Alexandria, he prepared a paper on gunshot wounds with his anaesthetist, Bill Alsop – 'upon which subject we rather set ourselves up as authorities!' – for which he was awarded a Hunterian Professorship. At his memorial service in 2003, reflecting on my father's distinguished career, one of his students, by then an eminent surgeon in his own right, joked that 'Aylett was known to have the fastest fingers in the business', something they attributed to his war experience. Beyond his personal ambition, however, by the end of the war he describes himself as 'vivid red' in his commitment to building a national health service which would be open to all and in which, ultimately, he would serve all his life.

Like so many fathers, mine spoke little about his war experiences, and like so many children, I missed many opportunities to explore them with him. When I read this book for the first time I was in my twenties, just out of university. From the first page I felt immediately exposed. This was the voice of a passionate young man whom I hadn't known. Its intimacy went beyond the unspoken boundaries which exist between parent and child and immersed me in the raw feelings of a man living through events whose enormity I had barely understood. As a child I had internalised this war unconsciously: in the home with my parents and through war films on television, and in public through memorial events such as the death of Winston Churchill, when my father took us to file past his coffin as he lay in state. However, as a young woman I stood at a critical distance, filled with a deep sense of distrust in the vested interests that had presided over this catastrophe and profited from it.

While he was preparing the book, my father did take me to visit Normandy. This was always an emotional heartland for him, alive with memories. On our way to a war cemetery, with a straight road stretching ahead of us, I remember risking the question, 'What did you know about concentration camps when they sent you to Sandbostel?' We were suspended in time then, the no-man's-land of flat agricultural acres stretching grey on either side of us, and he began to tell me, for the first time, about what he had found. There is a passage in his book when looking back to 1944 where he puts this experience in perspective.

> I had returned [to France] skilled and tough and tempered like steel in the heat of so many makeshift operating theatres. Nothing could shock or shake me now. No further episodes of war could hurt me as they had. Time was to prove me wrong. Work in a concentration camp was yet to come. Its stark, shattering horror lay in the future.

Among my father's documents, I came across a box: Letters Home, 1939–45. He had written to his parents almost once a fortnight, even if only a couple of lines to say he was alive and fit. Only the retreat from France in 1940 silenced him totally. It was testimony to the efficiency of the mail services, although letters to England arrived more reliably than letters between different war fronts. I probably owe my life to the fate of one particular letter which went astray. It was written to the nurse he fell in love with before sailing for Africa in 1940. It was delivered, then redirected, redelivered and redirected again. When months later it finally reached her, carrying his proposal of marriage, she had just returned from her honeymoon.

My father had included a handful of letters in his memoir and details from others he incorporated into the narrative. In this edition, however, I have added several more. In the compulsion to communicate events as they unfold there is the raw intensity, self-irony and wit of a young man trying to make sense of each day's adventure. He is less guarded, particularly in relation to his superiors, than he felt able to be when writing nearly forty years ago and the letters include stories which do not appear in the original.

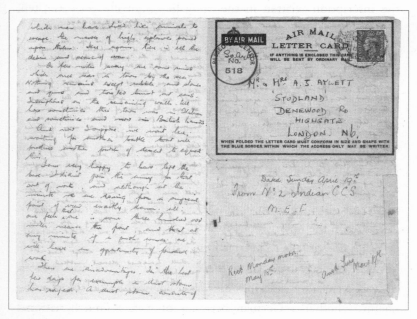

My father wrote every fortnight to his parents in London.

Most of the letters were marked with the date of reception in pencil in my grandmother's perfect handwriting. Reading them, I sensed my grandparents' hands on the thin, blue airmail pages and the huge emotion that accompanied that first reading; I imagined the discussions afterwards and saw them combing through details to track where their son might be, trying to match events with the news reports (names of places were not allowed by the censor), and always with the nagging doubt that he might not have survived the two weeks that had passed since the letter had been written.

I would like this new edition of my father's testimony, illustrated with his own photographs, to reach tomorrow's witnesses, not least through the digital platforms of the Internet. I also hope that generations to come will learn from it, and in the spirit of the inscription written in the copy he originally gave me, will recognise that 'to know a little is to understand much'.

War is an extended act of killing that, wherever it takes place, implicates us all. We partake of its ghastliness and hear its cries even from afar – from Central America, the Balkans, Rwanda, the Middle East, Iraq and Afghanistan in just my own lifetime. None of us can be immune to its consequences. Remarkably, my father's chronicle places us in the midst of appalling acts of destruction, but keeps us in touch with what is positive, a pulse of life, often with the sense of absurdity which sustains the human spirit through such times. 'It may seem silly,' he tells his parents in a lull between casualties in the desert, 'but I'm just off to play a game of football.'

What does it take to keep feeling alive in the midst of brutality? How do we stay true to our humanity beyond the polarisations of war? My father describes his ambivalence when caring for the enemy, whether a German prisoner of war, a French national serving in the German army, the old woman with whom he is billeted or the young German girls abducted from the streets of Bremen and brought in to help clear the concentration camp. He also expresses the human need to restore balance by focusing on things of beauty and harmony, whether in the arms of a lover, amid the monuments of ancient Egypt or in the daily laughter and companionship of his medical teams.

Sitting by my father's bedside that night in 2003, I was haunted by an unease which had pursued me for some months. I would have liked to phrase it as a question, though I knew it would have been impossible for him to answer. It had the face of the child, grown up, still yearning for the father's protection, for ultimate solutions. It was about how best to live, fully, the all of it. Recalling it now, I realise that in those last shared moments, my father and I were both facing a similar uncertainty, although at very different points on life's journey. In preparing this edition of his book, I realise that what he has written is, in itself, an inspirational part of the infinite answer.

HOLLY AYLETT, 2015

AUTHOR'S PREFACE

Throughout the war I was an inveterate diarist, using my own peculiar form of abbreviation. There were, of course, many occasions when entries had to be delayed, but eventually they were included. These I transcribed soon after my discharge from the army and these transcriptions coupled with innumerable letters I wrote, particularly to my parents, served, together with my memories, as the basis for this book, which I have now had the leisure to assemble.

Among all the war books little has been written concerning the Royal Army Medical Corps (RAMC), which was responsible not only for the good health of our soldiers throughout the zones of war in which diseases, often almost unknown in this country, were endemic and which, without preventive precautions, could decimate an army, but also, of course, for their care when wounded. The sooner such wounds were treated surgically the greater would be the soldier's chance of recovery and, with this in mind, the

Corps pushed its surgeons, their anaesthetists, nursing orderlies and nurses, when possible, as close to the fighting areas as was feasible.

This is a personal story, but more importantly it is an account of how our wounded were cared for and operated upon in the most difficult of circumstances close to the fighting, and as such it describes the experience of dozens of us forward surgeons.

With the very rare exception, none of us were consultants. We were what were then known as registrars – in effect, chief assistants in our departments. We all held a fellowship of one of the Royal Colleges of Surgeons, but most would have needed two or three years of further training before we would have been considered for consultant appointments.

Nevertheless, we had all been trained in the principles upon which success in surgery depended and these principles we applied. We had no experience of the surgery of war and little of trauma. Road accidents and major disasters were not common before the war. But the necessary and essential modifications to civilian practice we learned rapidly, and we would have been more adept than our seniors had they suddenly been called upon to take our places.

The provisions made by the RAMC alter in the same way as the design and strategy of war itself. What was effective in the last war will not be so in the future if nations, in their madness, ever engage in another worldwide conflict. I cannot envisage in the future a situation in which forward surgeons and their teams will be deployed as we were. Casualty clearing stations like ours would be too vulnerable in an inevitably more mobile war and instead a Corps fully equipped with helicopters with which to transport wounded from forward areas to surgical services miles away in the comparative safety of a base zone would be more practical. The delay in treatment would not be increased.

This book is, therefore, apart from an account of many incidents, the story of an era in the history of the Royal Army Medical Corps which is past but which remains a part of its proud and distinguished record.

STANLEY AYLETT, 1979

1

THE DAYS PRECEDING THE OUTBREAK OF WAR

SEPTEMBER–NOVEMBER 1939

I took my friend down to the barracks. The sky over London was fiery red. It was the glorious red of an evening late in summer, not the hideous cruel colour that even then must have been adding its light to the eventide falling on burning Warsaw. Early that morning we knew that the long wait had all but ended. The first editions of the morning papers, appearing then almost as soon as the last hour of the old day had passed, told of an impossible ultimatum made to Poland, and in the morning the headlines announced the first air attack of the Second World War.

It was as if we were watching a very sick man, who, nursed through all the precarious stages of a long and desperate illness, was being suddenly overwhelmed by a dreaded complication that put at nought all the endeavours of months of effort. For him only a few hours remained until the final crossing over, and for the world, too, there was but a little while before it plunged into unknown horror, suffering and death. Now the practice blackouts, which had attracted almost as many crowds to the West End as a New Year's Eve, and the unfamiliar barrage balloons, around which the gazers gathered in unhappy wonder, were to become a part of our lives. The khaki, navy and air-force blue uniforms which were so rapidly replacing civilian suits were no longer part of the unreality of an England living in so-called peace but were symbolic of the very things on which all hope was based.

That morning the everyday life of our hospital had ended. Green Line coaches, converted into ambulances, had filled the hospital forecourt and we had said goodbye to our patients as they left for their country destination. The hospital was empty – as empty as it had never been since the day it had first opened its doors decades ago. In the wards, filled only with their rows of clean white-sheeted beds, there was a quiet so uncustomary that involuntarily one hushed one's steps as if walking in a church. It was a quiet that was almost lonely. Blued sunlight streamed through windows painted as an aid to the evening blackout. At a large centre table in the ward a sister and her nurses were quietly cutting and packing tens of hundreds of wound dressings. Outside, sandbags were piled high. Stretchers were stacked and the operating theatres prepared. The hospital was ready should Warsaw come to London.

We went down to the common room. It was just before a quarter past eleven. The wireless was turned on. Neville Chamberlain's voice told us what we all knew was inevitable: we were at war with Germany. Less than a year ago a Whitehall packed with people had welcomed with relief his words, 'This is the second time in our history that there has come back from Germany to Downing Street peace with honour. I believe it is peace for our time.' Less than a generation ago the war to end all wars had come to a final armistice. We remained silent. As young doctors we were accustomed to arguing and debating any topic. But for this cataclysm there were no words, only each one's thoughts of the past and fears for the future.

Within minutes, it seemed, the sirens were pitching high and low. The first air-raid warning of the war. Was London so soon to be as devastated as Warsaw? We went to our allotted posts to await casualties. But none came, nor did they for weeks and months during that period of what became known as the 'phoney war'. In the days that followed, this great teaching hospital was at a standstill. Only a few essential emergency and accident cases were admitted and these were evacuated away from London as soon as possible. But as the expected air attacks failed to materialise it gradually reverted, albeit to a limited degree, to its customary function as a district hospital.

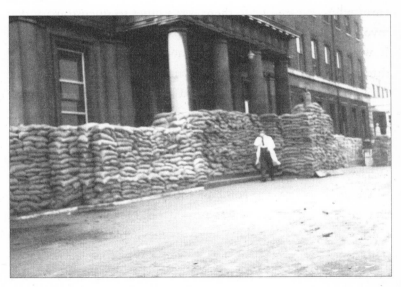

King's College Hospital prepares for war.

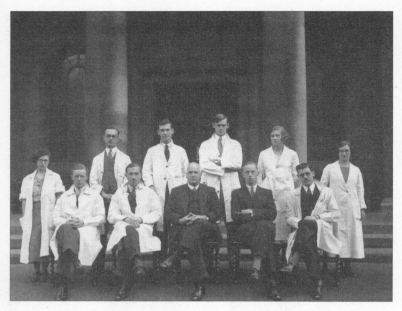

King's College Medical Team with the author in the back row, third from right.

A week after the outbreak of war, I was in the army and on my way to Tidworth. The London stations were crowded with mobilising servicemen and women. Once again after a lapse of little more than twenty years these cold bleak places were to witness the hopeless poignancy of parting and the radiant happiness of reunion. Mothers and fathers and wives and sweethearts were saying goodbye as I joined the train – and who knew if that goodbye would turn out to be their last? Theirs was the hardest part. They had to go back to houses where the empty room and the unoccupied chair could never let them forget – not for a moment – that a precious part of their lives had been wrenched away. They knew only too well what war was like, that it is filthy and evil and that it hurts and hardens. We, who were young, knew nothing of this. We did not know what war meant. We had yet to see the simple homes of innocent people lying in a confusion of bricks and mortar or the masterpieces of

4

man reduced to the elements from which they were raised. In the freshness of youth we had no idea how years of war would age us. It was knowledge of this that explained the unspeakable sadness and the tears that welled uncontrollably in the eyes of those who waved us goodbye.

I suppose that when I arrived at my destination I expected to find a unit bustling with activity in preparation for a rapid move overseas. Here was I, complete with brand-new valise, camp bed, basin and bath, riding breeches and leather gaiters, and all the other paraphernalia that only experience would prove unnecessary, but which I had been instructed to purchase. It seemed not unreasonable to suppose that the unit to which I had been so expeditiously sent would be similarly fully equipped. However, the actuality was very different. I had yet to learn that the wheels of mobilisation moved slowly in those early months of many deficiencies, and the unit I had come to join had progressed no further than obtaining a few bell tents and some cooking gear. Most of the personnel had not yet arrived and the only indication that this was a unit at all was a few officers gently settling down to an afternoon's siesta in the late summer sun. I knew at once that the sense of urgency conveyed in the telegram I had received was exaggerated. I could have lingered a few more days in London.

It was a pity, as experience proved, that the army used the word 'forthwith' with such carefree abandon, for familiarity with its so frequently unnecessary use bred a certain contempt for it. Now and then it really did have meaning, and by luckless chance these were nearly always the occasions when a leisurely day or two had been spent in clearing up or having a farewell party. Irate telephone messages were then required to speed you on your way and considerable ill feeling was generated. When the message read 'forthwith – repeat forthwith –', one knew one had to hurry.

There were other units around us in a similar state of

unpreparedness, and for want of something better to do with us authority decided that a little parade drill would be beneficial. So we were all assembled and marched away. Undoubtedly it is a mistake to parade a cross section of doctors of all ages and of all sizes, taken from general practice, from public service and from hospital and consultant life. It does not enhance the parade ground or the sergeant-major's temper and neither is it good for the discipline of line troops who, rapidly learning what is afoot, gather to watch the fun. The medicos all feel terribly self-conscious, far more than the greenest recruit; he at least knows that this is part of the process which he must endure to become a soldier, whereas the doctor bitterly resents something in which he has no interest, at which he knows he is going to be bad, and which he is certain will not make him better at his job.

A rather bedraggled line is formed on the command, 'Fall in!' Most do not know what to do with their hands and can see there is nothing else to do but slip them gracefully into their pockets. 'Parade – parade, 'shun!' and there is a long-drawn-out shuffle instead of the customary click. 'Right turn!' ends in half the parade facing one way and half the other. Both halves think that they must have turned the wrong way and quickly reverse about. There is then a lot of talk accompanied by muttered curses as to which way they should be facing, interurupted by the voice of the sergeant-major who, red though he may be and with blood pressure high beyond the limits of that which can be recorded, manages to exert enough self-control to limit his cry to, 'Gentlemen, gentlemen!' with tragedy and pathos in his voice. Then comes the question of numbering and of course there is the inevitable wag who must say, 'Ninety-nine.' Forming threes is very complicated; any of us who have been in the Officers' Training Corps at school only know how to do it in fours, and it seems lamentable that all this hard-learned knowledge acquired in our youth has to be discarded.

Eventually we start off across the parade ground, not very proudly but with a good seventy-five per cent in step. The about-turn inevitably leads to disaster, as some remember to take one step forward before completing this difficult manoeuvre, whereas others – well, they just about-turn. The first half of the return journey is occupied by the doctors trying to find out where they were before starting the about-turn and endeavouring to recognise a familiar face to the left or right of them in order to give themselves some degree of confidence they are at least approximately correctly placed. No sooner have they got nicely into line than the debacle starts all over again. No, parades like this are not a success.

Another parade of which we were not enamoured was known as 'stick drill'. The supposition was that you would be out walking with a swagger stick, with which incidentally hardly any doctor was ever seen, or else on a parade ground similarly armed, and would need to know what to do with the stick when confronted by a senior officer. It would be easy enough just to tuck the stick out of the way under your arm and salute in the usual fashion. But no. In the early days of the war, as in peacetime, such simplicity just wasn't good enough and the whole thing had to be done, according to an arcane and much practised ritual, by numbers, which the executor murmured noiselessly to himself, and of course on the appropriate step. This we regarded as all rather silly and would rather have learned how to build latrines in the field or been taught the many facts concerning field hygiene of which we were woefully ignorant but about which we were supposed to know a lot.

Some days later, the unit personnel of this embryo casualty clearing station (CCS) arrived. Except for the NCOs (non-commissioned officers) they had all been recently recruited. Tents were erected, stores were assembled and the unit started to take shape. I think that one of the most marvellous things the army

7

did was to improve the physique of the nation's youth. Here was a cross section of the community, mostly round-shouldered, thin, out of breath with the minimum of exertion, lacking in pride and confidence and bearing. See them again later in the war, fit and brown, muscles rippling, proud of themselves and their unit and so full of confidence. It was something that never failed to impress me as the years went by, but it was equally tragic that it should take a war to raise the nation's standard of fitness from C3 (the lowest grade of fitness) to A1. Good food, fresh air, hard work and discipline all played a part in this mental and physical change.

At that time I was put in charge of the physical training of the unit because, as a student and young doctor, I had done a lot of PT. Exercises I found natural and easy, these newly joined soldiers found difficult and sometimes, to start with, impossible. But the change to a better physique for everyone had begun. I was also in charge of route marches as part of this training. I am a tall person with a long stride and find it hard to adopt the prescribed length of step of a marching column. I remember taking an early march and we had not been going for more than a mile or so when a rather breathless sergeant who was at the rear of the column came running up. 'Excuse me, sir,' he said, 'but I think you are going a little too fast for the company.' I looked round and there trailing away into the distance were the men of the CCS I thought were at my heels. The heavy packs plus my rather long stride had proved too much for them on this sunny afternoon and they had given up the unequal struggle of trying to keep up. In a few months' time, however, they would be able to manage it no matter how far and fast they were led.

My stay with this unit, which subsequently did excellent work in Norway, North Africa and Italy, was not long. Although a surgeon, I had been posted on its strength as a general-duty officer, but when the error was corrected I was sent to the large military hospital at Netley, near Southampton. This old building, erected in the early part of the reign of Queen Victoria, was an enormous barracks of a place, notable for the fact that instead of all the wards being built to overlook the lovely Southampton Water they lay on the opposite side of the building. There was a very definite story, which seemed to have been passed on from generation to generation of the Royal Army Medical Corps, that the building had been constructed by accident the wrong way round. It seemed the only reasonable explanation to account for the fact that the corridors and cupboards and not the wards should overlook the Water.

There I saw my first battle casualties: soldiers who had been wounded in the unrest in Palestine. Many of these men had been disabled with minor wounds for many months. So rapid is the progress of medicine and surgery in wartime that had they been wounded a few years later they would have been healed in a matter of weeks. But in 1939 the sulphonamide group of drugs used to combat infection was at little more than experimental stage; penicillin had yet to be developed; the value of the immobilisation of limbs, shattered by gunfire, in plaster of Paris was not fully appreciated; and the technique of war surgery was yet to make its great advances.

Towards the end of November some of us were posted to Crookham, the base depot of the Royal Army Medical Corps (RAMC), and two days later we sailed for France. The journey across the Channel might have been almost a peacetime trip, the ordinary cross-Channel boat having more civilians aboard than troops. The war seemed very unreal and far away, as it was to remain for all the months ahead, until May 1940 came and broke the spell.

2

SETTING UP HOSPITAL IN NORMANDY, FRANCE

NOVEMBER 1939 – NOVEMBER 1940

The 'phoney war'; setting up No. 6 General Hospitaloutside
Le Tréport; visit to Paris; a German agent befriended

The packet boat seemed to sail into the very heart of the town of Dieppe, as the port penetrates deeply into its centre. We berthed at the end of the main street. There were few signs of a country at war, except for some uniforms, a number of army trucks and ambulances and some blued-out windows. We disembarked and inhaled the so-different smell of France – a mixture of Gauloise cigarettes, perfumes and perhaps of drains as well. Along the waterfront the fishing fleet was preparing to go to sea. Nets were being stowed and stores and boxes taken aboard.

I had come from England with an anaesthetist, Major Frank Blackburn, as we formed what was known as a 'surgical team', a new component in the structure of the RAMC. Each consisted then of only the two specialists who, supernumerary to the staff of any hospital or casualty clearing station to which they might be attached, could be moved from that unit to any other more heavily engaged without disrupting the parent unit's capabilities. We had no transport, no surgical or anaesthetic equipment; nothing except our two selves. As the war progressed it became very obvious that to function adequately the original teams would have to be enlarged considerably and the highly successful field surgical units, or FSUs, were the outcome. Each FSU was provided with two three-ton lorries and a staff car and was equipped with tentage in which to set up an operating theatre and a small ward in which a maximum of twelve wounded could be nursed, although in practice this number was often almost doubled. Full operating, sterilising and anaesthetic apparatus and instruments were carried, and all the necessary drugs and dressings, beds, blankets and the like were stored in the lorries. The personnel consisted of the two officers (surgeon and anaesthetist), two drivers and seven other ranks of the RAMC in the charge of a corporal responsible for assisting in the theatre. This self-contained unit could be sent to any forward field ambulance or CCS and in less than two hours of its arrival, a ward would have been erected, an operating theatre set up and the unit prepared to deal with any type of battle casualties. But that all lay in the future and for the present we were but two.

On reporting to headquarters in Dieppe, located in one of the hotels on the front, we were told that we were to be attached to No. 6 General Hospital close to Le Tréport on the coast, some eight miles outside Dieppe. There, with others bound for a similar hospital, we were taken. For most of us this was our first sight of the Normandy countryside – fields cultivated to the very roadside, meadows green and lush, orchards growing apples for Calvados, gentle hills and sparsely scattered villages. The road went down a winding hill into Le Tréport, like those which wind down to so many of our small fishing villages in the West Country. At the bottom of the hill were the same narrow streets where the brown sails and the fishing nets were spread out to dry. At first it seemed the same as at home but then one noticed that the houses were more gaily coloured and that the fishing boats, too, had gaudy slashes of colour absent from those back across the Channel. I suppose this town in normal times, like so many in England, would have remained deep in its winter hibernation until the spring sunshine brought its first trail of visitors escaping from the cities. But this year, because of the war, as in the last when it had also been a hospital centre, it was dispensing with its winter sleep and there was a happy welcome wherever we went.

Our own hospital was a mile or so outside Le Tréport at a small village called Mesnil Val – at least that was where the hospital was going to be, for as yet it was merely a site. There was nothing except the personnel of the unit, who were billeted in the village. It was similar to the first unit to which I had been posted. A small hotel had been taken over as the officers' mess but it was full and there was no room for us there. We were lucky, however, because we were billeted instead in a wonderful *auberge*, the Hostellerie de la Vieille Ferme. This beautiful, centuries-old *hostellerie* was run by Madame Jean and her daughter whose husband was in the French army.

In the months till we left in May, Madame Jean looked after us as if we were her sons. Nothing was too much trouble. In the hard winter of that year when some of us had colds or flu it was not our doctor colleagues who cared for us but Madame Jean. She was an expert with mustard poultices and cupping. The latter treatment I had heard of but never seen, let alone experienced. Up to two-dozen so-called cups are used, each similar to, though more substantial than, a sherry glass. Into each a piece of cotton wool moistened with methylated spirit is placed and is then ignited. The cup is then quickly inverted and placed on the patient's skin wherever the inflammation is sited. In the case of bronchitis, which was my complaint, the full twenty-four cups are placed on the chest and kept on for about a quarter of an hour. As the oxygen in each cup is burned by the flame, a vacuum is produced and the skin is drawn into the cup. At the end of the session one is left black and blue as the suction ruptures the small blood vessels in the skin. Whether the cupping did the trick I do not really know, but because of it or in spite of it my troubles were resolved. The treatment was accompanied by the most wonderful invalid food, which made any discomfort it occasioned well worthwhile.

This hostellerie became for us far more than a billet – it became almost a home in which we were happy and at ease. Here in the evenings we struggled along with our limited French, some making more progress than others. We found ready teachers and helpers and each week as we improved we came to realise that the boundaries that separated us from our Continental neighbours were barriers easily broken down with knowledge and understanding.

For the older generation of this village the influx of hospital units was not new. Twenty-five years ago a similar invasion had taken place and the concrete foundations of previous hospitals still remained close to the cliff's edge as a reminder of those days. Up the hill was a large military cemetery and there lay those who had died in those units during the First World War. There was sadness and loneliness here, where the wind sighed and whistled among the orderly rows of beautifully tended graves. Here there was only one form of headstone, the same for brigadier or private. Here the commander lay at rest side by side with his sergeant or one of his soldiers, all equal in death. Beside any site that a large medical unit has occupied in wartime a cemetery is always left behind to tell of those who failed to survive the barbarities of war. Perhaps there had been peace for a while but at present it was hard to take into account. Somehow we had broken faith. Somehow all that had been bought at so great a cost was once more in danger. We had not been vigilant enough in the intervening years and now were being called upon again to defend what these men had died for.

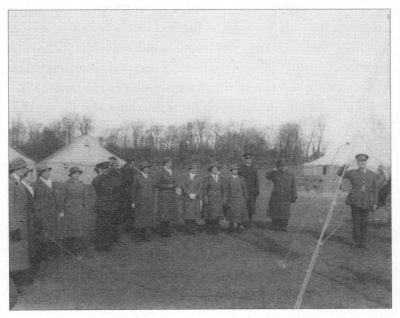

Dedication ceremony of No. 6 General Hospital, 1940.

Little by little our hospital took shape, slowly because equipment took weeks to arrive and we were inexperienced in the erection of the large and heavy marquees that had first to be laced together before they could be put up. We took great pride in their appearance. Each peg had to be in perfect alignment; not a crease in the canvas indicating a faulty guy rope was permitted. Each line of tents stood dressed alongside its fellows as perfectly as a company of guardsman on parade, and if one was not perfect down it came to be put up once again. We had yet to learn what it was to be under pressure in those early days; in later years a hospital such as this would be assembled in a matter of days whereas we took months. True the pegs would not have the perfection of alignment that ours had, true the marquees would look shoddily pitched compared with ours, but they would serve their purpose just the same. But now there was no shortage of time and as this hospital was going to be there for the war's duration it was going to be as good as we could make it. Who could have foreseen that before the summer came all of France would be overrun by German troops? In truth, the time was not wasted for we were learning all the fads and fancies of the hospital marquee, which were as many as those of a mule, and at the end of it all we were its masters. We could lace a number of them side to side, arrange them in blocks, put them end to end; in fact, do everything that could possibly be done with them. Unknowingly we were storing up precious knowledge for use in the years ahead when in a matter of hours our tents had to be pitched and the operating theatre ready for use.

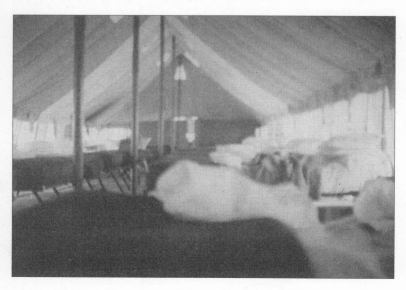

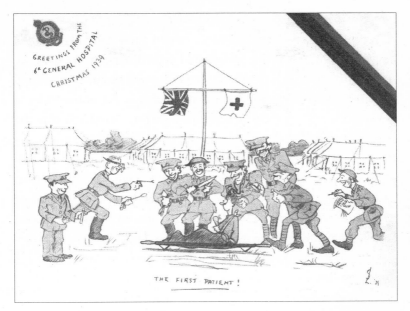

Christmas card, 1939.

That first winter of the war was severe and the ground often so frozen that the stakes split as we tried to drive them home. For a time, work on the hospital had to cease. At times the village was cut off and drifts of snow and iced roads made it impossible to use vehicles. We were kept busy looking after the sick there and in the scattered farms. The local doctors had been conscripted as soon as war had been declared and the nearest medical attention upon which people could call was often miles away, separated from them by roads, which were impassable.

For those of us who loved France it was a chance to understand and know its ordinary people better. We were always accepted with great kindliness and hospitality and we learned how terribly afraid these people were of what course this war would follow. Underneath their pride in the army they seemed to know that all was not well, that it was ill-equipped; that its leadership, politically

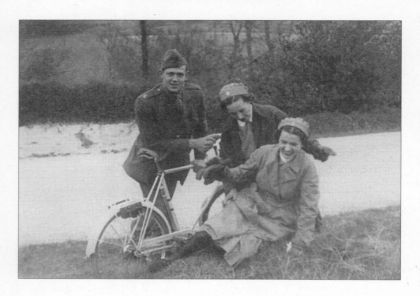

and professionally, was indecisive and divided. They were not frightened in the sense of wanting to run away but they lacked confidence in the power of France, even with its allies, to hold the Boche. What organisation there was did nothing to allay their fears. Air-raid precautions in England even in those early days were in a high state of preparedness. They bore no comparison to those in France, where they seemed to be almost non-existent. The blackout was not enforced and air-raid shelters were often the cellars of small houses with nothing substantial on top of them. There seemed to be no first-aid posts, no organisation for casualties and, of course, when the blitzkrieg did come, this lack of foresight exacted its toll.

One day about that time when the snows had disappeared, a young girl from the village was cycling down the hill when her brakes failed and she crashed into a stone wall. Her skull was fractured and spicules of bone had penetrated her brain. We were able to help. In an improvised theatre the wound was cleansed and the bone fragments removed. Happily her recovery was complete. The news travelled widely and prestige was high for No. 6 General Hospital.

April 2 – Major S. O. Aylett RAMC, No. 6 General Hospital, Headquarters Medical Base, Sub area, BEF

My dear Mum and Dad

Thank you very much for your parcel.

I'm writing this letter on a table I made myself sitting on my little camp stool, and on the other side of the tent is a chest, not quite in the Chippendale tradition, but nevertheless serviceable and also home made. I've got a couple of crates, a few duck boards and odd boxes. So it's not too bad.

I'm pleased to report that my dislocated elbow is now quite well. I've finished with rugger now forever, though the accident would not have happened had we been playing on a decent pitch. I caught my foot on a bump in the ground whilst going flat out and just went for six. I did not want to play but you know what it is, that you have to pull your weight in helping to prevent the troops from getting bored and to a certain extent to gain their confidence and that sort of thing...

Close by us is a big forest absolutely one mass of violets, primroses, anemones, cowslips and all sorts of other flowers. By the way I don't think I told you but I've bought a bicycle and any spare hours, we have cycling parties into the country. We have a rather steep hill close by and one of our favourite pastimes is a race down this. I expect one of us will have a spill one day, but it's one bit of excitement...

I think I'd better send some of my clothes home in case I have to move hurriedly, but we're still waiting patiently for something to happen hoping sincerely that it will, but I'm not sure that it is going to in the near future...

Well good night to you both.

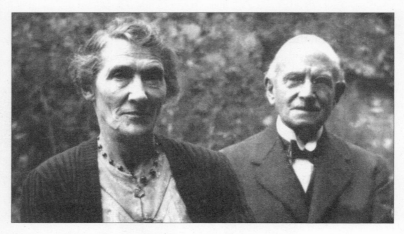

Arthur and Hannah Aylett in Highgate, North London.

Spring came to this lovely part of France, tipped the tree buds with green, yellowed the fields with cowslips and blue slips. It was as if nature for the last time before the holocaust was determined to dress in her best and look her loveliest. Some days we cycled down lanes where the fields were being tended right up to the grass verge of the gravelled lane, by the old and the womenfolk because the young had gone. Sometimes we walked to famous inns, to select the trout in the pool and to discuss with the patron the other food we should eat and the wine we should drink when we came to dinner on the following evening. Such a dinner was no sudden affair to be treated lightly but something to be pondered over and planned. Now and again we went boar shooting with our French friends in the Forest of Eu surrounding an ancient château. It was once owned by La Grande Mademoiselle, niece of Louis XIII and cousin to England's Charles II. Here they, too, had hunted two hundred and fifty years before. Here also, Queen Victoria had driven when, as a guest of Louis Philippe, she had stayed in the château.

Such an occasion was always exciting, not only on account of the hunt itself but because of the extreme wildness of the shooting. Along one of the wide drives that traverse the forest, the guns were stationed at intervals of about fifty yards and the boars driven by beaters and dogs down this gauntlet. But though all had strict instructions from the master of the hunt to keep to their allotted positions some were apparently dissatisfied with their own and crept gradually down towards the next station. When the boar rushed by, discretion was overcome by excitement, and as likely as not there would be a blast from just behind your shoulder as someone let loose at the rapidly moving beast. The British guests were not entirely immune from this rather Gallic fault, and on one occasion a very angry scene developed as a colonel accused a young major of nearly shooting him. We had to drive back some twenty miles in the same car after the shoot was over, and it was a journey completed in stony silence. The colonel never forgave the offence. A butcher always accompanied the hunt and at the day's end the boars were cut up, the various joints numbered and lots were drawn for each. Cooked in white wine they were excellent.

Paris is not far from Dieppe and I was given a weekend's leave to visit the city. Paris, striving so hard to be its beautiful and carefree self, half-heartedly preparing for a war that, desperately, it hoped would never come. The streets were darkened at night but innumerable glimmers from thousands of semi-blued-out houses and apartments must have been visible from the air. The towers and buttresses of Notre Dame were traced against the moonlit sky, and at the other end of the city the massive bulk of the Arc de Triomphe sheltered France's unknown warrior and the ideals of peace and home and love of which he had dreamed.

The hotels were overcrowded but I was lucky to be lent a room in a flat which belonged to a girl I had met in Mesnil Val. Every bistro and bar seemed to be filled to capacity. Theatres were packed and uniform predominated. At the Casino de Paris was a two-star spectacle with Maurice Chevalier and Josephine Baker. Their songs either tore at the heart or made love seem to be a thing as natural and sparkling as champagne. For a time the memory of that evening lingered; the magic of it all was reality, with the world outside merely a stage peopled by soldiers, sailors and airmen.

★　★　★

Another short leave period was spent in London. I arrived unannounced but was given a wonderful welcome. I soon realised that my father, to whom I was very close, was worrying about something and I got him to confide in me. The cause of his concern had its beginnings in the late twenties when my brother Arthur, who was then at Cambridge reading modern languages, went to stay with a family to perfect his fluency in German. It was an exchange visit and the following year the family's son, Hans, came to stay with us. He was a pleasant young man, studying engineering at his university, but perhaps seemed slightly effeminate with his perfumes, powders and aftershave lotions with which we, at that time, were quite unfamiliar. He told us of the tide of National Socialism which, under the then almost unknown Adolf Hitler, was starting to sweep across Germany. Although he was not associated with the party it was apparent that its ideals had his sympathy, a sympathy shared indeed by many prominent English men and women. Hans became almost one of the family; he visited England on many occasions over the years and always stayed with us. He never avowed membership of the Nazi Party but his support seemed greater each time. During the daytimes he disappeared ostensibly to explore London and its surrounding counties but we never really knew where he went. One thing about which we came to be surprised in these later years was that at a time when currency export from Germany was under the tightest control, Hans never seemed short of money.

I think it was towards the end of 1935 that he rang to say he was staying at Bishop's Stortford and that he would like to come and see us. This was odd because, as far as we knew, he had never stayed anywhere but with us on his numerous visits to England. Nevertheless we were delighted to hear from him and when he called we not unnaturally asked what he was doing. He told us he was supervising the development of an air brake that, somehow, could check the steep descent of an aircraft and allow it to come out of its dive without losing its stability. It appeared that an English engineer, working for a tyre factory in this country, had evolved the idea and had offered it to the British government. Failing to arouse any interest, he had then taken his blueprints to a department of the German government, which, in contrast, showed marked enthusiasm. The engineer was asked to stay in Germany to work on the project but he did not wish to leave England for any long period of time. It was therefore agreed that Hans, representing the department concerned, should supervise the initial stages of the development in England. This would have seemed a normal procedure but the workshops in which it took place, and which we were to visit, were anything but normal.

We asked Hans where he was working and he told us, rather vaguely, that it was near Ware. My brother then enquired as to whether we could come and visit the place and, perhaps with some reluctance, Hans agreed to take us. Late one afternoon he drove us to a small café, in quite an isolated spot, on the Cambridge road outside Ware. In a field behind, and unseen from the road, were some newly erected sheds. We had tea in the café and at six o'clock it closed. As soon as the last customer had left lights came on in the workshop and lathes started to hum. Hans took us over. I asked why they only worked at night and he told me that there were two reasons. First, they were working on a secret invention and the less people knew about it the better. Secondly, the English engineer worked in a factory during the day and it was only at night that he was available. It seemed a reasonable explanation. But as I looked at the steel discs gripped by lathes in various stages of turning, some spoiled and discarded and others lying on the benches, I did not realise I was looking at the prototypes of air brakes for the Stuka, the bomber which was to terrorise so many cities and armies in Europe. I did not see Hans again. After about six months he returned to Germany. We went again to visit the café and the workshops, but they were closed and shuttered and becoming derelict.

My brother met Hans for the last time in early 1938. Hans said then he was sure that a war was inevitable and that he would like to have some money in England as he thought it would be safer, giving the impression that he believed Germany would lose. He asked my brother to invest this for him. It was a strange request, but they were friends and Arthur took the money and invested it in some British bonds. Later that year he wrote to say that he would like to stay with us again and we arranged to meet his train. However, he telephoned from Harwich to say that he had been prevented by the immigration authorities from entering the country. Our last contact with him was a letter my brother received a few months before the outbreak of war, saying that he was leaving Germany and was going to North America, whether to the States or Canada he did not say.

My father then told me what had happened to worry him. 'Two days ago,' he said, 'the telephone rang and I answered it. On the other end was a man who, although he spoke perfect English from a grammatical point of view, I am sure was not English. He had a trace of an almost guttural accent. He asked whether Arthur was there. I told him no, and he then asked where he could contact him as he wished to collect the money which had been loaned to him by Hans. I said that I had no idea where my son was and that I certainly knew nothing about the money to which he referred. At this the caller became aggressive and said that I must know where my son was. As he grew heated his accent became more pronounced and I am sure he was a German. I hung up on him. Now, in view of all our associations with Hans I wonder whether I should tell the police.'

I told my father that in his place I would do nothing unless the call was repeated; least of all would I write to Arthur about the incident in case the letter was censored. I explained that if the letter was opened by chance by the censor, Arthur, then serving at sea with the Royal Navy, might be suspected of collusion with the enemy. In the event my father had no further telephone calls.

Why should Hans have wished to invest money in this country when he must have known he was going to America? Why, when in England, had he always seemed to have as much sterling currency as he wished? Why had someone tried to obtain the money he had left with my brother? I understood my father's worries as to whether, quite inadvertently, we had befriended a German agent. Later, when Arthur was serving on one of the corvettes escorting a convoy out of Halifax, Nova Scotia, which lost seventeen ships, I again wondered.

During that leave I visited old colleagues who were working in the Emergency Medical Service which had been set up at the outbreak of war, but a certain coolness had developed and a gulf seemed to separate us. It was an understandable reaction. We in the RAMC were not doing very much while they at home were working hard, with staff numbers reduced by our absence. Indeed, one of my senior chiefs suggested that he should apply for my release from the army as I seemed to be wasting those skills I possessed and would be far better employed working at my old teaching hospital. I declined his offer. I had joined the army and I intended to serve with it until the war was over. I was very happy to return to France to rejoin my unit.

Our nurses arrived in early spring. We welcomed them at the hostellerie. They looked efficient and lovely in their grey suits faced with scarlet, the uniform of the Queen Alexandra's Imperial Nursing Service, and we knew that we had the best nurses for what was going to be the finest army hospital in France. We danced that evening. It could have been peacetime. Only the uniforms and the records we played – 'Run, Adolf, Run, Adolf, Run, Run, Run' and 'We're Gonna To Hang Out The Washing On The Siegfried Line' – ill omened as they were, reminded us we were at war.

From then on the hospital came alive. Stores and equipment poured in. The operating theatres became real, the pathology department had benches and microscopes, the X-ray tubes were in place and wards were filled with beds, white with sheets and red with blankets. One of the heaters, great fat stoves we called Goerings, was installed in the centre of each marquee, which had now become wards. Outside the entrance to every ward a bright garden had been planted and we vied with each other as to which should be the best. Orderlies, nurses and officers, all were proud of the hospital and, within the hospital, of the unit to which they belonged. It was beautifully sited in the fields at Mesnil Val, surrounded by orchards which were then a mass of blossom, white and pink. We would at least be able to offer our wounded a setting of peace and loveliness, away from the filth and horror of battle.

So the springtime passed and the blossom dropped from the apple and cherry trees and one night the silence was broken by the noise of aeroplanes. It was 10 May, and the period of the 'phoney war' was at an end. It had been called the phoney war because in those first few months there was no reality, nothing, not even the sureness of battle or of death. What lay in the future no one knew and from the past we were uprooted. There was just our small world which was tangible and for the present very sure. Things that seemed so certain back at home were far away and it was only now that mattered. There might never be a return to the life and the world which had ended the previous September. Sufficient to live in the present, and to live the present to the full; to forget about the past and not to think about a future that might never come.

As news of the German invasion came through, Major Blackburn and I received orders to proceed as a surgical team towards Belgium. We packed our bags ready to move. The hospital had been a very happy one and we were sorry to say goodbye. We had learned much, particularly from the CO of the surgical division, Colonel Frobisher. A regular serving officer in the RAMC, he knew everything about laying out an efficient operating theatre in a tent. He had learned all the little tricks somewhere in Mesopotamia in the First World War and these he willingly passed on to us. However, he could never reconcile himself to modern methods of transport. 'It would never go on a camel,' he would say, sadly looking at an enormous steriliser or a giant packing case, and obviously pondering whether it could be slung across some poor animal's back. He missed his camels and would have been far happier loading a ship of the desert than supervising the packing of a three-ton lorry.

3

THE GERMAN
BLITZKRIEG ON BELGIUM
AND FRANCE

MAY–JUNE 1940

*My first casualty clearing station near Lille; in forward areas with
No. 159 Welsh Field Ambulance in a convent near Ypres,
then a school kitchen, also in Belgium; back in France with CCS
at Steenvoorde; retreat towards Dunkirk and escape from beach
in abandoned motor launch; rescued from sinking craft by
HMS Havant; return to Dover and RAMC depot*

An ambulance took us eastwards towards Belgium. We drove
through the beautiful Forest of Eu with its vigorous new
growth green and shiny in the early summer. Bluebells and
anemones carpeted its open patches. But as we reached Arras and
beyond, the big trees seemed to fall away and there was nothing
left save the tangled scrub of the last twenty-odd years. There were
ominous craters and mounds, unnatural ditches all clothed in a
verdant green to hide their one-time ghastliness and horror. We
passed so many patches of 'England', with row upon row of silent

stones, patches where the dead were no longer to be allowed to sleep in peace.

Daylight passed and the hundreds of lorries filled with stores and troops, ambulances, transporters and guns crawled now northeast towards the border without lights, the drivers feeling their way in the darkness. In the distance there were lights but they were not the innocent signs of habitation, but the glow from burning buildings or the occasional, too occasional, flash of ack-ack (anti-aircraft) guns.

We arrived late that night at a casualty clearing station just outside Lille. It was sited in a large house that had previously been a home for incurables but was now set up as a semi-permanent hospital, which would have been ideal if the circumstances of the First War had prevailed. Already the ambulances were pouring in with their wounded and soon the floors of the wards were packed tight with stretcher cases. With ourselves there were three surgical teams and we started to operate at once. The unit became hopelessly overcrowded and yet still more cases came. In the later years of the war, when the organisation of the RAMC had become first-class, when the doctors and personnel had increased in numbers sufficient for most needs, there were few occasions when the amount of work was beyond the capabilities of the unit. But in the campaign in France it was quite impossible ever to get on top of it.

The opportunity of evacuating cases to a hospital at the base so that they could receive treatment there rapidly ceased. Disorganisation of evacuation facilities set in at an early date. Roads were blocked by transport and columns of refugees and strafed by aircraft. Ambulances could not get through and as often as not were themselves the objects of attack from the air, in spite of the Geneva red crosses painted on their roofs. Within a few days evacuation by train had ceased. Some hospital trains had run into stations only to find they were occupied by the Germans; others were rendered useless by the destruction of the railway tracks. Evacuation of patients would be planned, only to be cancelled at the last minute, and in time ceased altogether. Every corner of the floor space was occupied. Row upon row of touching stretchers. Men pale and weary, their clothes filthied with mud and dirt, stiffened with drying blood around torn and jagged entry wounds, lay there for the most part quiet and silent. Their splints and bandages hid the remains of torn-off limbs, and bony ends covered with earth stuck out through lacerated skin and muscle. Sometimes it was only when a bandage was removed that the full extent and sickening sight of some awful wound revealed itself, guts flooding on to the stretcher canvas, gaping, ragged holes in the chest that poured blood as soon as the pressure of the dressing was taken away. And above all was the smell of sweat and faeces, of exposed flesh decaying. Almost with fear you removed the bandage from a man's head, wondering whether you were going to see eyes, swollen and sightless, or to see a hole pierced in the skull from which the brain oozed and almost dripped. What a feeling of thankfulness and relief surged through one's heart when a wound was only superficial. It could not have been worse at Scutari or Gettysburg, even though here we had the most wonderful skilled nurses to help us.

We had hundreds of patients but we could only deal with the most severely injured. In this respect the surgeon was always up against a grave dilemma. From a manpower point of view it was obviously of the greatest importance to return as many men to the field as possible and to keep their stay in hospital and their period of convalescence to a minimum. This was logical and reasonable and according to this logic we should never have operated upon the man hanging between life and death. There was no doubt that when treated early the period taken for a wound to heal lessened appreciably and the soldier returned to his unit far earlier than if allowed to go untreated for some days, especially in that first campaign when we were short of sulphonamides and penicillin had not yet been developed. The wound suppurated and took weeks to heal. From a military point of view those were the cases we should have operated upon, but we could not do this and instead took to the theatre only those whose condition was desperate. We knew that many stood a poor chance of recovery even if treated by urgent surgery. We knew that if nothing were done they would surely die.

Many hours were probably wasted because, in spite of everything, a fairly high proportion of these wounded did die. But was the time really wasted? Some did not die. Some defied the laws of probability and recovered, and although we may have delayed attending to the more lightly wounded this was justification enough. An example was a soldier who had gas gangrene of his foot. Gas gangrene is a deadly enemy of the soldier wounded when fighting in the well-manured fields of the Continent. The organisms abound in the soil and readily invade grossly damaged tissue; once there, they multiply and grow rapidly, producing toxins which kill the local area and poison the patient with toxaemia, Apart from the appearance of the wound, which may be black and green and bubbling with gas, the presence of the infection can be recognised by its peculiar odour. A nauseating, heavy and revolting smell hangs in the air of a room in which lies a victim of gas gangrene. The leg of this infected man was amputated below the knee and for two days he improved until the gangrene started to invade his stump and progress to his thigh. His only hope was a further amputation just below his hip joint. The operation was performed and against all the odds he recovered and returned to England, where he was fitted with an artificial limb. He happened to be one of my cases, but any of my colleagues would have done the same. They, too, had operated on patients whose recovery astonished and encouraged them.

In the Middle East gas gangrene was rarely seen because the

organism did not flourish in the uncultivated desert sands. Later on in the Normandy campaigns, penicillin came along to control this terrible complication of war wounds, but in the British Expeditionary Force in 1940 the infection was rife.

Conditions of work became more and more difficult in this clearing station as the days and nights went by. With all of us at full stretch there was no time to restock and to prepare the hundreds of dressings we required, let alone to sterilise them. This latter probably made little difference as every wound was so contaminated. The theatre became increasingly dirty after hours of operating and a brief respite had to be taken to wash it down with disinfectant. Then gauze would be hastily cut. In the rows of wounded we had to separate the urgent from the 'can wait' cases. Transfusions had to be set up but blood was at a premium. We slept little and ate when we could.

All around our CCS the desolation and despair of war intensified. Most of the French in the northern areas seemed to have lost confidence in the ability of the Allied armies or of the Maginot Line to contain the Germans. Many of them had bitter memories of the previous war when they had suffered occupation by the Hun. Now, often in their old age, they pictured it all returning, the shambles of war, the fabric of their lives lying in ruins, and they were afraid. It was a sense of blind escape that urged them in their thousands to crowd on to the roads without thought of where they were going as long as it was westwards. On farm carts overloaded with furniture and bedding and all the possessions of a home abandoned; in wagons drawn by weary horses or even pulled by hand, with the very old and very young nodding in disturbed sleep; on bicycles and on foot all laden with parcels and bundles, this pitiful and tragic stream filled the roads. The columns moved on, silent and hopeless, with mask-like faces, dogs and farmyard animals with them, too exhausted to move out of the way of army transports. Troop movements were slowed and the confusion was added to by air attacks. The wounded were brought in to us. There were no other alternatives.

For the first time we were seeing war and it was cruel and harsh and evil. We could try and repair its ravages but nothing could restore two arms to a little French boy, nothing could bring back the sight to the blooded eyes of a small girl, and nothing could bring hope to a young French wife whose womb was a mass of flesh torn apart by machine-gun bullets. Our senses became dulled and that was just as well because, in spite of all, we had to keep going.

I do not think any of us then had any idea that the campaign in France was on the verge of disaster. We talked in the confident manner peculiar to the uninformed of how, even if the Germans did break through Belgium, they would be held at the fortified line running across the north of France. That lay reassuringly between us and the border, so we thought, and it was only later that we were to discover it consisted in places only of wagons and farm implements laid across the road to stop the progress of the Panzer divisions.

About this time we had a royal casualty. HRH the Duke of Gloucester had been caught in a severe bombing raid near Tournai and both he and his aide-de-camp were more than lucky to have escaped with nothing worse than lacerations, with which we quickly dealt. In some way it seemed that the enemy had knowledge of his whereabouts. He had only left Arras a short time before his billet there was bombed, and his car had also been attacked from the air. Undoubtedly there were many exaggerated rumours during these weeks about spies being at work, but that a lot of fifth-column activity was going on was beyond question.

★ ★ ★

All of the confidence we had in the future was suddenly shattered. We learned that Arras had fallen, that a further German breakthrough had occurred and that they were now almost upon us. It was decided by the administration of the Medical Service that the CCS could no longer admit casualties on account of the difficulties of getting them there and of the impossibility of evacuating them. Our own surgical unit and one other were therefore ordered to take equipment and move forward to No. 159 Welsh Field Ambulance. Two ward sisters accompanied us. This proved to be an administrative error, but happily the correction did not catch up with us until we were near Ypres and had already undertaken heavy periods of operating. Then we were told that the nurses had no business being up with us so far forward and they were promptly removed. When they went we missed their skilled help, ceaseless and seemingly untiring beyond measure. As the war progressed over the years the ordinary man in the street who had joined the RAMC became increasingly highly trained in the technical work of the Corps, which included nursing care, organising the theatres, sterilising the instruments, preparing the operating equipment and even assisting at the operations. But at this time most of them had not had sufficient experience to carry out these duties with the efficiency of our nurses and their recall was a serious loss to us.

We found No. 159 Welsh Field Ambulance already dealing with the wounded in part of a convent and within an hour and a half of our arrival we were operating on our first case. For nearly thirty-six hours we worked, only stopping briefly for cups of tea or pausing when the theatre was such a shambles of dirty dressings and blood that we had to stop to bring a little order out of the chaos.

That night I remember well because we nearly had a serious fire, which could have involved the whole building. All our heating and sterilisation depended, as was the case in the forward units right until the end of the war, on Primus stoves, and the care and maintenance of these – and if they are going to function efficiently they need very special looking after – was sadly neglected in the RAMC. One of the stoves had been continually giving trouble and when it finally went out one of the orderlies, attempting to light it again and forgetting that the burner was red hot, poured some paraffin into the igniting cup. French paraffin is more like petrol in its inflammability, and the stove and the paraffin container instantly burst into flames. The fire rapidly spread to the blackout curtains and other equipment in the theatre. We were operating in a wash-house and only because of the availability of water were we able to get the fire under control. There was a wounded man on the operating table and ether in the bottles around the anaesthetist. With dirty black smoke over everything, we bore little resemblance to men in white coats, but disaster had been avoided and after briefly clearing up, we went on operating.

May 22 159 Field Ambulance, BEF

Dear Mum and Dad

This is the first unit I've been with. Everyone keen, good and out to help each other in every way. I haven't changed my clothes now for four days, worked a 24 hour shift the other night and most hours the rest of the last 10 days.

We operate in a big room. Conditions are bad but we do our best. We set up a theatre in an hour from absolutely nothing, start to operate and in the 24 hours I was on, I and another chap did 50 each. I just fell asleep in my clothes, but the unit as a whole received a congratulatory message from the Big Noise. I must get back to work again

With love from, in the circumstances, your very contented Stanley

That was our only session in that convent. We cleared up, prepared further dressings for our next spell and fell asleep for a few hours fully clothed. We were awoken to be told that we were to move at once into Belgium. We packed our stores hastily and loaded them on to a lorry. The convoy of vehicles, of which our lorry was one, edged its way towards the border on roads clogged with human traffic and through villages whose streets were barricaded with carts and wagons, allowing hardly room for a lorry to get by. We crawled along, often held up completely by the westward-moving mass of refugees, unconsciously helping the Germans by hindering the forward movement of the British Army. As we approached Belgium the roads became clearer and the houses were empty. Sometimes we passed tank traps and barbed-wire entanglements we knew to be hopelessly inadequate against the mass of steel that was descending on France.

We crossed the frontier through what had once been a busy and prosperous town, but which was now divested of its civilian population. Shuttered windows, empty streets, an occasional scared dog vainly seeking its departed master, were all that greeted us. Even the frontier itself, which divided Royal Belgium from the Republic of France, no longer had any significance. The gates were wrecked and open, only the red and white poles remained pointing aimlessly towards the heavens.

Again we were struck by the growth of everything. Houses and trees had grown up all around that town where the Allies had held on during the last war. They were in harmony because both were young. Here old age did not exist either in nature or the designs of man. Sadly, the life which had so recently sprung up anew was also destined to be uprooted as history repeated itself.

This time we set up our theatre in the kitchen of a school. In our previous location we had had the advantage of electric light, but here we had to rely on acetylene flares, and when periodically these faded out, we completed operations with the aid of electric torches. We worked on, losing count of hours, even of days. Now and then we ate and slept, but there was no respite except for the briefest of periods. The wounded came, it seemed, in a never-ending stream, and there were no other forward surgical centres close by to relieve us. There was no alternative but to go on and on until we were almost overcome by sleep as we operated. In this respect the anaesthetist was in an enviable position as he was sitting down and could snatch from time to time a few precious minutes of oblivion.

Around us the bombers were meting out destruction against resistance which seemed negligible. Flying low, hedge-hopping sometimes, they came at will to select their often innocent targets – the red cross, whether on ambulance or train or hospital, was not always a guarantee of sanctuary and protection. Our nursing sisters were discovered and ordered back to base. We were glad they were going on account of their safety, but sorry as they had been of such enormous value and help to us. They had given our impromptu theatres a businesslike air, which disappeared with their going. They had had so much to do with the organisation under difficult circumstances and when discipline slackened it was their encouragement that improved and maintained it. We missed them very much, but they went with the knowledge that no other nurses had served so far forward or indeed with a field ambulance.

Soon after, with the falling back of the Allied troops, we too were on the move again. Lorries were hastily loaded, the remaining wounded evacuated in ambulance cars and the journey back began.

While in the school we had taken a liking to a small deal table which was extremely useful for putting our dressing drums and instruments on, so we decided to take it with us, but as soon as it was obvious the unit was on the move some nuns, who apparently ran this school, appeared as if from nowhere and eagle eyes were cast over each article that was carried out from the building. They fell upon the table and, eventually, in spite of our pleading, back it had to go. No doubt the Germans found good use for it.

We crossed back into France, along roads crowded as before. Fear was now adding itself to the despair of these wretched refugees, giving added impetus to their flight and driving them on when physical weariness and mental fatigue bade them lie down and rest. They saw the retreating armies. They knew the reason for the retreat.

At this time no one seemed certain of the position of the enemy troops and one cheerful subaltern of a famous artillery regiment with whom I made enquiries said, 'Well, sir, we have been shelled from over there, from over there and from over there,' pointing roughly to the north, south and to the west, 'so presumably they must be there; but of course it's quite possible that the shelling is coming from our own batteries.'

We attempted to set up a surgical centre again but machine-gunning, bombing and near shelling made it obvious that we could not work there long, and at this juncture we were detached to join a CCS working a little farther back at Steenvoorde.

So we said our farewells to No. 159 Field Ambulance. It was a Welsh territorial unit and for efficiency and cheerfulness in all circumstances one that would prove hard to beat. No one worked harder than its commanding officer. He scarcely slept for days on end, organising and encouraging during that difficult period. I well remember one morning, when we had a brief breakfast break, how very tired he looked. As I watched he started to bring a fork up to his mouth, but in spite of himself his head nodded, his eyelids drooped and as he slumped back in his chair fast asleep the fork dropped from his hand. We were all closely approaching that stage.

There was no accommodation for another theatre in the CCS to which we were sent, so we had to share one that was already set up with another surgical team attached to the unit. From our point of view this was fortunate as it meant that we had periods free from operating in which we could sleep. There comes a stage when it is useless to carry on without a rest and we had to give into it.

For a few days we worked there, aided in the nursing of our patients by a band of French girls who had stayed to do all that they could to help, but the town was on an important crossroads and was the frequent focus of enemy bombing. Another CCS working in the same town suffered a direct hit with the loss of some of its patients and several of its personnel. This time, however, one could not blame the Boche as the medical units were sited too close to a legitimate military objective.

At this CCS we became really conscious for the first time that the situation was becoming desperate. There was uncertainty everywhere and the stories from the wounded of how their units were being overwhelmed by the Germans and countless supporting tanks was ominous. Around, many fires were burning where the Stukas had dived and now bursting shells were close. My anaesthetist and I were given orders to proceed in the direction of Dunkirk and to rejoin No. 159 Field Ambulance. We were given a map reference. We had no transport, but there was no difficulty in that respect – on the roads were many lorries whose drivers had either lost their units or had failed to reach them in places where the Germans had broken through. Many of these men naturally enough did not know what to do and were more than pleased to attach themselves to some unit and to be given constructive orders once again. We therefore stopped two empty lorries and having ascertained that they were completely lost we loaded our wounded and our equipment and set off.

We could not avoid a feeling of depression because it seemed that after such a short time the BEF (British Expeditionary Force) was facing far more than a minor setback. Everywhere the roads were barricaded far more heavily than before, and in the distance it seemed that thunderclouds were gathering on that hot summer's day. Little did we realise that what we thought were thunderclouds a few miles away was actually the smoke from a burning Dunkirk, but as we drew nearer the truth dawned. On the road we were told that the main approaches to the town were blocked, that we were to report at Bergues for further instructions and, worst of all, we learned then that the whole BEF was being evacuated back to England. It was terrible and shocking news. It hardly seemed possible that we were being driven out of Europe; that the Hun was winning wherever he chose to strike. We knew that things were going badly, but none of us had till then doubted that somewhere in France a line would be held. We were appalled by the news.

On arrival at Bergues, we were told to leave our wounded there and then to rejoin No. 159 Field Ambulance; we had not finished unloading when this little town on the way to Dunkirk was blasted from the air. As we left, what had been a few minutes before an old walled town of great beauty was now fast becoming a smoking ruin.

From here to Dunkirk, as the roads converged towards the port, was an army in retreat and it was a tragedy to see the army of one's own country edging back towards the sea. Behind us now was a half-circle of infantry, armoured units and gunners, protecting this retreat and delaying the enemy advance to make feasible the evacuation of the majority. Units were marching back towards a port on fire. Lorries trundled northwards to take their loads as near the point of evacuation as was possible, and straggling along, saddest of all, were parties of weary, dirty and unshaven men, many of them wounded, whose own formations had been scattered and broken up. It was an army that had been beaten, not because it was lacking in high morale and confidence and courage, but because it had not had the weight of steel to pit against a fully armoured enemy.

We searched vainly for No. 159 Field Ambulance just outside Dunkirk, but they were nowhere near the rendezvous that we had been given, so we went on towards the town hoping that we might pick them up there.

I suppose that as we approached that blazing town, overhung by a pall of smoke that blotted out the summer sun, there was not one of us who did not experience a mounting sensation of fear, however much we may have disguised it. Lorries and transport of all descriptions now lined the sides of the road in confusion. Some were burned out, some broken down, others driven over banks into ditches and waterways in order that they should not fall intact into enemy hands; there were others, their drivers crumpled and huddled over the steering wheel, which had been machine-gunned or bombed by the attacking Luftwaffe. Everywhere there was a feeling of frightfulness and doom, and the cold grey waters let loose to flood the countryside in an endeavour to hold up the advance added to the depression of it all. Elsewhere the sun was shining but here it could not pierce the evil smoke of desolation.

The air in Dunkirk was hot and reeked of burning. It seemed that not a house stood that was not damaged or on fire. Overturned and wrecked lorries and trams and ambulances littered the streets in a scene of total devastation. Raiders dived low shooting out of the smoke clouds above, to the accompaniment of the stabbing noise of machine guns and the shrieking howl of falling bombs. We leaped from our lorries on these occasions and rushed for shelter under cars, under the screen of a wall or even against the bole of a tree.

On one occasion, I crawled under what seemed a substantial-looking lorry and I remember being quite surprised to find myself the only occupant of such excellent cover. When the raid had passed and I had crept out, a driver came towards me. 'That's a fine place you chose, sir,' he said. 'It's my lorry and I left it in a hurry. It's full of ammunition!'

We sought once more unsuccessfully for our field ambulance, hoping to find them as we were useless on our own. We had been instructed to leave our surgical equipment behind with the CCS and without this we were of no more value than a gunner would be without his gun. We could do practically nothing for any wounded. It was only with a unit that was set up and functioning that we would be of any use and we decided to travel back again towards Ostend in the hope of finding one. None of us could see any possibility of evacuation; we were sitting targets for the attacking planes and only a miracle could rescue us.

We went eastwards along the canal, always listening with one ear for the near approach of enemy aircraft and always ready to make a dash for the nearest ditch as the roads were sprayed. Often we would fall on top of some other soldier who had beaten us to it, or someone else would come toppling in after us.

We crossed into Belgium again through a deserted frontier post. There did not seem to be many troops around now and most of those there were Belgians wearily trudging towards the border. The ones we spoke to had little idea what was happening, had heard vaguely of a capitulation of the Belgian army and were hoping to escape to France and then to England. While we were enquiring, an RAMC officer in his truck came down the road. He was with the Blood Transfusion Service and told us that he had tried to reach a unit in Ostend but that the town was already occupied by the German army; he advised us to turn back. So once more we crossed back into France. We stopped at Coxyde, a small town just across the border a few miles outside Dunkirk and filled to overflowing with refugees of all types and descriptions. Everyone anxiously asked us questions. Were all the army being evacuated?

Could they come with us if possible rather than be left in the hands of the Hun? Did we know what all these rumours of a Belgian capitulation meant? Hundreds of questions were showered upon us but we knew the answer to none of them. All around us was anxiety, uncertainty and fear of an awful unknown. We could do nothing, only wait as we had been told that some further evacuation might be arranged from the Coxyde beaches the next day.

Any hope of escape for the entire BEF must have seemed desperately remote, with the circle growing hourly smaller, but nevertheless spirits rose when we spotted the RAF again weaving and circling round the Luftwaffe. As we saw our tormentors shot out of the sky, with all of us on the ground excitedly cheering, we felt that somehow some way would be found out of this impossible situation.

That night we slept in a room at the very top of a hotel, far too tired to worry about whether it might be hit during the night. There comes a time when fatigue overrides all coherent thought.

As dawn broke we were up and could see, lying grey in the early-morning light, the silhouettes of destroyers and transports anchored off the shore already embarking troops. We found a divisional headquarters from which we obtained definite orders to leave, but by that time the ships had filled and were creeping out to sea. A cruiser remained, firing broadsides into enemy positions, and then it too crept silently away. Somehow one's heart sank as this link with England – we were not to know it was not the last link – faded into the distance, while over the coast the drone of planes and the flashes of gunfire ushered in a day of continuous air activity.

Later three drifters appeared and beached on the high tide. One was filled with petrol, one with ammunition and one with food and general stores. These were to be unloaded when the tide receded, and they would then be used for embarking troops.

At least that was the idea, but implementing any such organised programme was out of the question. All that day wave after wave of bombers and fighters came over, the latter often just skimming the beaches so that one could see the faces of the pilots. High explosive and incendiary bombs and machine-gunning precluded unloading and soon two of the drifters were on fire and the ammunition was exploding.

Now and then an attempt would be made to unload the remaining drifter carrying stores. A party would leave the sand dunes that lay above the beach to cross some quarter of a mile of sand down to the ship, and then inevitably the Luftwaffe would dive. There was a desperate race with death, with half scattering towards the sea and half towards the dunes with the sure knowledge that only speed could save them. Always there were a few who hesitated and that hesitation was often fatal. We collected the wounded and carried them into the sand dunes and did our primitive best for them, improvising splints and applying dressings to wounds.

Sometimes fighter aircraft would come almost skimming the tops of the dunes. We could see their approach and we would bury ourselves on the side of the dune away from the plane. Then, as the pilot wheeled to return, a small army of men would rise up and leap down on the opposite side of the dune as once more the bullets sprayed. We got quite expert at this game of hide and seek; there were few casualties and the wounded were well protected. Many of the soldiers blazed away at the planes with their rifles. It was good for morale but I doubt whether it caused the pilots any concern.

With evening a severe thunderstorm came to our aid and the planes were driven from the sky, but by this time the tide had flowed in and the surviving drifter was nearly floating. The ship was feverishly unloaded into the sea and a stream of men then waded up to their necks to climb the rope ladders to get aboard. The shore was littered with gear and equipment of every description, except the rifles to which nearly every man clung. And among this equipment the incoming tide gently lapped and caressed the bodies of those who had died that day.

Our number of wounded, many desperately ill, had increased during the day and the only hope for some was to get them back to England as soon as possible. I went down to the water's edge and waded out to the drifter to see whether a dinghy could be launched to pick up the worst cases so they could be brought out and loaded on to this ship. I was up to my chest in water as I shouted my request. A lieutenant-colonel came up to the ship's railing. He was berserk and pulled out a revolver and I looked straight into its barrel. He told me to get back and that none of the wounded were going to be taken aboard. He was so completely out of control that I knew he would shoot me if I persisted and so I waded back to the shore. The drifter filled up and sailed. Another link with England had gone.

I rejoined Major Blackburn at our first-aid station. We decided what to do. First, we, along with our driver, smashed our lorry. With hammers, iron bars and a pickaxe we made sure it was one vehicle the Germans were not going to use. We then went to look at a motor launch that we had previously noted high up on the sand dunes, a reminder of the previous summer's peacetime days. As we looked at it we were wondering whether we could get back to England in this 'round the bay in the *Skylark*' type of boat. It looked dry and old, but at the time there seemed to be no alternative; it was a case of trying to cross the Channel in this or remaining to be captured. We could not move far from the beaches because of the number of wounded for whom we were now responsible. Perhaps somehow we could drag the boat down to the sea and make the crossing in it.

By this time there were many more troops arriving – Belgian, French and British – and in addition a sergeant pilot who had baled out that morning. He played with the engine of the boat while we looked on anxiously and then, to our delight, it roared into life. If only we could move it down to the sea we stood a chance. We immediately set to, straining to push and even lift it down from the dunes. It seemed an immense distance to the sea although high tide was approaching. Then out of the skies once more the enemy planes dived and we sheltered as best we could.

Little by little the waves came in and foot by foot we edged the boat towards them, hoping that the tide would not recede before we reached the surf because we knew that it would ebb far faster than we could hope to push towards it. We tugged with all our strength until at last the bows were lapped by waves and cheered as we strained and felt a shudder pass through the boat. It must float now, and the tide was still not quite full. We loaded our wounded, then exerted one last mighty push as a larger wave came rushing in. The boat floated and shot out into the sea.

The beach must have shelved at this point because suddenly all of us who were pushing were floundering, struggling and swimming in deep water. I remember so well the face of a Belgian who had been toiling at my side; with his enormous physique, a bristling square-cut red beard and on his head the old-type helmet of the Belgian army, he had been a tower of enthusiasm and strength. But he could not swim and suddenly he was struggling for dear life. I remember seeing him carried away by the tide, roaring, gasping and still fighting hard. I hope he managed to reach the shore.

In this unexpected confusion I was somehow able to grasp the side of the boat and hung on until someone hauled me aboard. I was by then far too exhausted to climb in by myself. All around were troops floundering in the deep water, and many of them drowned. Some we managed to drag into the boat, but of those a few, although they had only been in the sea for what appeared to be a matter of moments, died in spite of all our efforts with artificial respiration. I suppose the exhaustion of days without sleep, as well as the heavy clothing that the troops were wearing, had something to do with the quickness of these deaths by drowning.

The motor once more roared to life and we started off across the Channel. As the shore of France became more distant and the buildings blurred in the twilight, an overwhelming sense of failure swept over one. Three short weeks of war and we had been driven out of Flanders and the north of France. Like the thought or not, the ugly reality was we had been beaten and the future seemed dark indeed; victory now seemed almost impossible. We were leaving behind France and its people, whom during the months we had been there we had learned to respect and understand. Some of us too had left a part of our heart behind, there on the continent of Europe. The fear, the excitement – yes, even the thrill of the last few weeks – were being replaced by emptiness and depression. We felt that we had failed. We were all very tired, of course, which didn't help.

We made our wounded as comfortable as possible, but a poor standard of comfort it was with the sea coming over them in fair quantities and soaking them as they lay on the deck. They never murmured. They never uttered so much as one word of complaint, and for them it must have been so much worse than for us who were at least unscathed. Three of them died. Someone forced a prayer book into my hand and I read a brief service over each before we committed them to the sea. The bodies did not sink but drifted away, drawn by the tide to the shore on which they had been mortally wounded. Violent death had become our close companion in the past three weeks and it had come to stay it seemed. But we knew it now for what it was. It had no glory in it;

48

no peace and loveliness. It was evil and cruel and so sad that there were times when one wept.

The summer darkness fell as we chugged uncertainly along. We were still a long way from home when, to make matters worse, the boat, dried by being out of the water for so long, began to leak; then the oil in the engine ran out and we found ourselves drifting and wondering how long it would be before the boat sank under us. We were not alone; we could make out other small boats, some so laden that the bigger waves lapped over them. In the distance was the reddened sky over Dunkirk.

After a little we could distinguish the silhouettes of destroyers in the failing light. They signalled to us as they passed so that now, even though they were hurrying away over the horizon, we felt sure that we would be picked up, and sure enough not long after another destroyer came towards us. So closely packed with troops was this ship that it could only take off our wounded in addition to a few others and the remaining twenty of us waited to be picked up by a further destroyer, HMS *Havant*, returning from Dunkirk.

The thrill and relief of finding myself on the steel deck of a warship bound for England was indescribable. All the pent-up nervous tension of the past weeks suddenly vanished and desperate tiredness took its place. I wanted to sleep and sleep for hours and hours. Nothing else now seemed to matter. Every inch of the deck space was crowded with exhausted troops and down below the between decks were crammed. Yet somehow or other hot cocoa was served to everyone by the ship's company. There are some unforgettable things in this world and that cup of cocoa will always be among them for me.

We landed at Dover, stumbling across several ships' decks before we reached the quayside. Why these ports of disembarkation were not bombed by the Luftwaffe is hard to understand. It was surely a major blunder on Hitler's part, because the chaos such attacks would have produced could have been immense. The crowded troops, the ships moored side by side, the constant flow of trains arriving and departing provided ideal targets. Mercifully they were left alone.

Some hand of genius must have organised the train services that sent the hundreds of thousands of troops who arrived from across the Channel to all parts of England. Trains came in, they were loaded quickly and as soon as they were filled they drew out. Had there been months of planning behind it, the clearing of the ports could not have been more efficient. I followed the line of troops towards the train, clutching the bar of chocolate and the apple which each of us had been given and feeling rather like a tired small boy coming home from a picnic and bringing the remains of the high tea with him. There were a few brief minutes in the train devoted to eating our food and then the precious oblivion of sleep, undisturbed until our arrival at Aldershot.

We drove through the morning sunshine to our reception camp. England seemed almost unreal in its accustomed and unchanged peace; it did not seem possible that a few hours' journey away men were not walking to their day's labours but were engaged in a desperate last stand in which it was a case of kill or be killed. It did not seem possible that so close at hand the sky was filled with danger and death while here only the birds sang in the heaven of early summer. No journey on a magic carpet could have produced such a change in so short a space of time. We had come back from another world but one which would encroach on this island's shores soon enough.

We were taken to the RAMC depot at Crookham, given break-fast and then told to proceed to our homes on leave as best we could. Because a succession of other trainloads of troops from the Channel ports were on their way to the various depots in England, these had to be cleared as soon as possible. It was difficult to clean the mud and dirt and the salt and blood from our uniforms, although they were given a superficial sponge. Saturated and filthied tunics needed more than that to make them presentable once again and the surprised glances of our fellow passengers in the train to London made us realise that we were not as spic and span as officers of His Majesty's Forces should be. But we were too weary to worry and anyhow we were going home for a few days' leave and before us stretched the prospect of hours and hours between clean white sheets. I eventually knocked at the door of my parents' house and saw all their anxiety and foreboding well into relieved tears at the sight of me. I slept for eighteen hours.

4

CREATING A
HOSPITAL AT DOVER

JUNE–SEPTEMBER 1940

From Leeds to Dover and a false alarm

Within a few days a movement order came telling me to rejoin No. 6 General Hospital, now in Leeds. This was the hospital unit I had left at the beginning of the German Blitz and it was starting to re-form and re-equip. It had been evacuated from the west coast of France but every bit of its equipment had been abandoned in the fields close to Dieppe. It was to be months before once again it was ready with all its specialised stores, tentage and surgical requirements. The whole of the personnel of the hospital were billeted with families living in the vicinity of our assembly point and the hospitality and kindliness of these Yorkshire people knew no limitations. I, myself, was in the house of Mr and Mrs Butler, whose family business was Kirkdale Forges, and I was looked after in the manner of an honoured guest.

Meanwhile, England was preparing to repel an invasion and

Dover was to be one of the outposts of the country's defence. After a brief stay in Leeds, I was sent there to organise some sort of hospital arrangements for the garrison of the western half of Dover mainly sited in and around the Citadel, an old fort that dated from the days when another master of Europe was casting covetous eyes across the Channel. The eastern side of the town with the great castle as its centre was to be provided with another hospital.

If Dover were to be cut off by an invasion on its eastern and western flanks, which at that time seemed a high probability, it would be quite impossible to evacuate casualties, and in each of the two small hospitals the wounded would have to be accommodated and given surgical and medical attention for a matter of weeks. But neither hospital existed, and myself and my counterpart at the castle, Major R. Isaac, each had to create one. Neither of us was even given an anaesthetist, but I was fortunate in that the RMO to the Royal West Kents, who were garrisoning the Citadel, was seconded to me and he had had considerable experience in this field. I was given seven medical orderlies but they were raw in the extreme with the barest knowledge of nursing. It seemed extraordinary that with so many skilled personnel available, for example those attached to the hospital I had just left who at the time were doing little, we should have been provided with so little help. We were very critical of our senior officers at Maidstone who seemed to have no appreciation of what the proposed projects entailed.

Out of nothing we had to achieve something. We had no quarter-master or administrative staff and the business of assembling the hospital equipment, laying in stores of rations, surgical dressings, anaesthetics, drugs and the host of other necessities which would be required if we were cut off for two weeks or so, was our responsibility. In spite of the difficulties it was a job full of interest. There is always a thrill to be had out of building or creating something where previously nothing existed.

To use as my hospital I was given the basement of a large building used as the officers' mess of the Royal West Kents. It was piled literally feet high with the debris and dirt and filth of many years and this, as a start, had to be cleared out and the whole building washed and scrubbed again and again. Medical officers on occasions have to be scrubbers, tent pitchers, stretcher-bearers, painters, lorry drivers and a host of other things, and this was one of those occasions. Arrangements had to be made for electric lighting, independent of the main supply, as it was highly likely that the latter would be cut; for fitments to be made to the theatre; for water tanks to be set up; and for all the equipment for this small hospital to be obtained. There were no definitive stores from which the latter could be acquired and high and low we scoured the Dover area for beds, mattresses, bedpans, bottles, pyjamas, paraffin stoves and the many other essentials necessary even for a modestly fitted small surgical hospital. It was one of those times when nearly everybody helped and the indent orders and red tape were reduced to a minimum save on a few memorable occasions.

We had been instructed to have the unit ready to function at the earliest possible date. I contacted the area officer of the British Red Cross with a view to obtaining certain medical comforts and other hospital accessories. The lists were filled in and forwarded to her office. However, they were returned requesting that the signature of the Assistant Director of Medical Services should be obtained. The forms were immediately sent off to him with a request that, in order to avoid further delay, he sign them and forward them direct to the Red Cross. Nothing happened for over a week when, instead of the expected stores, a red-hot letter came from this officer's department. What right had I, it asked me, to contact the Red Cross before first obtaining the permission of his office? Moreover, in future I must not contact his office direct but must go through the normal channels via the Senior Medical Officer,

Dover. The lists were returned and the latter's approval would have to be obtained before we could have the sanction of his office for the supply of these requirements.

At this time there were certain incompetent cherry-tabbed officers who resented any enthusiasm among those recently commissioned to act with independent thought, but these, fortunately, were few in number. In the event, the supplies I had requested did not arrive until weeks later, due to these quite unjustified delays. Further trouble with this masquerading incompetent came over the question of nurses. It became obvious very soon that our orderlies were insufficiently trained and lacked the experience necessary to give a severely wounded man every chance of recovery. At that time Dover was being shelled as well as bombed and the casualties, although not numerous, were often severe. We pleaded to have two nurses attached to our unit, but nothing would make this man see reason. Why he was so against giving us nurses I never understood. Perhaps because he hadn't foreseen the need, he disliked his lack of foresight being brought to his attention. His statement that Dover was no place for nurses when there were ATS and Wrens in large numbers held no water with us.

One night, after a particularly severe period of shelling, we were hard at work and a severely wounded man died. Perhaps even with first-class nursing he might still have died but we felt otherwise and decided that a protest must be made against this refusal to give us efficient nursing help. To any doctor the loss of a patient, if some stone has been left unturned, is a disaster and something with which he reproaches himself. We felt this way about this soldier and appealed to the consulting surgeon. He agreed entirely that there was a crying need for nurses, and advised the senior officer accordingly. Red in the face to the point of apoplexy, he refused to budge and no nurses were sent.

Fortunately we managed to find an ATS officer who had been a trained nurse. It was thanks to her work in her off-duty hours and the help of a naval sister that we were able to improve the comfort and treatment of our patients. But it was not through official channels that this improvement was achieved.

At the beginning of the war there still remained a few combatant officers who regarded the RAMC as a burden rather than a benefit, as an encumbrance rather than as serving any very definite and useful purpose. As the war progressed this misguided opinion was dispelled completely, and apart from any other consideration, the boost to morale that troops obtained from the knowledge that not far away was skilled surgical and nursing care was fully appreciated. Divisional and Corps generals knew that the disposition of their medical services was as important in a battle plan as the siting of their guns.

In Dover, however, a certain battalion CO still adhered to the old school of thought with regard to army medical services. Though charming and friendly, he could never be accused of being fully cooperative in medical matters. It seemed to him so much waste of space to have a lot of hospital beds about the place when the space could be so usefully employed for storerooms, offices or training rooms, in fact for anything but a hospital. So he thought – until the day arrived when he was forced to change his mind.

The Luftwaffe was at that time using a new form of cannon shell, numbers of which failed to explode. In Dover it was a very strict rule that if any were discovered following a raid, they were to be moved only by the bomb-disposal units, on account of the fact that a large number had exploded on being picked up. It so happened that at the end of an air attack the colonel came across some of these shells scattered on his parade ground and being of an enquiring turn of mind decided to remove some to the armoury for dissection. As he was carrying them away, however, one of them went off. Although more than a little shaken, he was not so much concerned about his fingers, which were a bleeding mess with the tips hanging off, as that this injury, sustained as a result of a very obvious and open breach of orders, should not be reported on any official form. Such a small oversight in our report books caused us no misgivings, and as in addition the colonel's fingertips, sewn back into position, survived most satisfactorily, we had a strong convert to the viewpoint that far from being encumbered, the battalion was very fortunate in having a hospital within its lines. From that day forward there was never any difficulty in acquiring added accommodation or extra help for the unit.

Dover was very much a front-line town in those months when the prospect of invasion hung heavily over the country. Scarcely a day passed when, out of the sunshine, squadrons of yellow-nosed Messerschmitts did not swoop on the town, first destroying as many of the balloons as they could and then spraying with their remaining shells whatever objective took their fancy. Then would follow light bombing attacks, and as the warning time was of the briefest, Dover was continuously on the alert.

It became the centre for newspaper correspondents, for newsreel men and even broadcasters recording for the first time the sounds of war on England, sounds that were to become even louder and more menacing in the years to come, sounds that were to disturb the peace of country hamlets as well as make themselves heard above the roar of the great cities. Houses had started to topple and death was coming from the sky to the housewife out shopping and the child racing with his playmates in the streets. Shopkeepers were having to sweep up the glass from their broken windows and householders were learning to extract their treasured possessions from heaps of rubble. It was the overture to the second act of a tragedy more full of sorrows than any before written, and Dover had the best seats.

From the other side of the Channel periodic flashes of flame could be seen as a shell was fired across the sea, and a hundred seconds later the air would reverberate with the sound of a high explosive bursting out of its eleven-inch casing. Through the narrow strip of water that separated the free from the fettered world, ships still steamed up and down, slowly, steadily, as if unperturbed by the fountains of sea that were being thrown up all around them by the bombs and shells. As closely as possible they hugged the friendly English coast, sometimes enveloped in a smoke screen laid by protecting warships. But this was a gauntlet through which they had to pass. There was no escape from it and they chugged through its narrow confines watched by countless anxious eyes from this town on the front line of the free world.

In the evening the correspondents gathered to eat and drink and talk at the Grand Hotel on Dover's front (until one day some of them had to be dug out of its ruins). Then when darkness had fallen fully the roar of RAF machines on their way to attack the massing invasion forces on the French coast signalled the rising of the curtain on a fairyland of lights and colour twenty miles away, while the windows in Dover trembled in concert with the boom of distant explosives.

Rumours of impending invasion were rife, and at times they were more than rumours. One weekend in September a telegram arrived from a high official source. It stated that according to reliable information received, the invasion of England was due to start on the following day – a Sunday – at 3 p.m. Dover developed into a hive of industry. Lorries roared through the streets and up the hills on either side of the town, in and out of the Citadel and the castle, transporting troops, stores, ammunition and light equipment. Additional guns were towed into their new positions, while the population of Dover watched with worried faces. This was obviously no ordinary scare they thought; this was the real thing. In our hospital everything was ready. The sterilisers bubbled, the reception room was clear, the resuscitation room was lined with bottles of plasma and saline. Outside the ambulances stood by.

The weather was perfect; a hot shimmering haze lay over the Channel. I suppose everyone was trying to discern beyond that haze the thousand massing barges that would bring the invasion for which we waited. Three o'clock passed into four o'clock and the minutes slowly ticked away till five. Then a further telegram came which simply stated: 'For England read Indo-China.' It was the day the Japanese had decided to march into the former French possession and somewhere a mistake had crept into the initial message. Dover relaxed once again into its normal routine of daily air attack and occasional shelling.

We were proud of our little hospital, which in spite of all the difficulties managed to fulfil its function reasonably efficiently. Cooking for and feeding sick patients was one difficulty, but with enthusiasm and a Primus stove a lot can be done. Some of our orderlies developed into very reasonable cooks and into nurses of a good standard. It was a unit of such small numbers that everyone was very important and there are few people who in such circumstances will do anything less than their best. We were therefore a little disheartened by a senior brigadier who arrived one day as a patient.

Although our hospital was intended for the treatment only of battle casualties and the few sick who were likely to be in for short periods of two or three days, an exception was made in the case of this officer who wished to remain in the Dover area and did not want to be evacuated. We prepared what we considered a very reasonable room for him – even went to the lengths of staining and polishing the flagged paving floors and buying a bunch of flowers to put on his bedside table, but I think he must have believed he was going into a London nursing home because from the start nothing was right. One morning after we had been up all night dealing with urgent shelling casualties he sent for me to complain that not only had his breakfast been served late but the porridge had been cold. There are times when patients' complaints are reasonable but this one was so unjust that, brigadier or no brigadier, the position had to be explained in very definite terms and he had to understand that when there were desperately wounded patients in the hospital even a brigadier's breakfast might have to be delayed a little. He was man enough to apologise but the link of faith that binds patient to doctor had been broken and we were pleased to see him go.

5

ORGANISATION OF THE RAMC

OCTOBER–NOVEMBER 1940

No. 6 General Hospital, Luton; to London
for course on tropical diseases

About October of 1940, the Luftwaffe started to change its tactics. Previously its attacks had been concentrated on the numerous airfields in the south of England in an endeavour to destroy the fighter squadrons, but this plan had failed and the bombing of the big cities, with London as the first objective, commenced. Daily the blocks of bombers passed over the coast around Dover to be met first by an ack-ack barrage, which strove to break up the armadas, and then by a fighter formation. Many got through but the daily toll was high and the victory rolls of our fighter pilots were a common sight against the blue skies of autumn days.

Notwithstanding the barbarous nature of this new development, some units of the army still seemed to offer an attitude of outdated chivalry to the bomber crews who had been shot down. I remember one prisoner who had been captured by a neighbouring unit being given a bottle of wine with his evening meal and on a visit I made to an army hospital I noted that each German, although only lightly injured, was served beer with his lunch, a luxury our own wounded did not get. Those of us who had seen civilians being machine-gunned on the French roads by the same air force had a certain idea of the type of mind we were confronting and we had no such misguided feelings of chivalry.

As early winter came the prospect of invasion, at least for that year, disappeared and I was ordered to close our small hospital and to rejoin No. 6 General Hospital, now in Luton. Here it and a similar unit were busy mobilising for service overseas, assembling and packing all their equipment, checking, numbering and detailing it so that delays would be minimal when the hospital came to be set up.

The Royal Army Medical Corps during the last war had been faced with a formidable task made the more difficult by the rapidity with which battles advanced or receded in the new age of mobile warfare. From that war of 1914–18 it had learned many lessons, administrative as well as technical, but these had to be changed or modified as a result of the experiences in the brief battle of France from which, in spite of most difficult circumstances, it had emerged with credit. The organisation of forward surgical units, so that urgent life-saving surgery would be available to the soldier within a few hours of the receipt of his wound, had yet to fully evolve, but the concept of the big base hospital to which casualties would finally be evacuated and their treatment completed remained.

At the outbreak of war few, if any, of the great cities of the United Kingdom had hospitals provided with a thousand beds. Yet in all theatres of war were to be found such hospitals, some capable of accommodating even two thousand patients, with resources enabling them to offer practically every type of treatment that a great hospital at home could provide. There were special units for nervous diseases, for head injuries, for plastic surgery, for specialised facio-maxillary restorations after gunshot wounds – indeed for all eventualities – in addition to those concerned with general surgical and medical care. The actual accommodation was only a part of the challenge. All the wards, laboratories, operating theatres and offices had to be lit and large generators with all the wiring necessary were carried as part of the equipment for this purpose. The maintenance of efficient blackout under tented conditions, the laundering of thousands of sheets and towels, overcome by providing mobile laundries, and the adequate provision of cooking facilities were all problems that were associated with a general hospital in the field. Then, when the soldier was recovering, departments for his rehabilitation, including skilled physiotherapy and every form of massage and electrical treatment, had to be available.

In whatever part of the world the army was involved, these hospitals had to be set up. Each had to carry with it the accommodation in which to nurse its patients, provide quarters for the personnel – doctors, nurses and other ranks – install specialised laboratories and X-ray units and operating theatres. In certain areas local buildings might be used or a civilian hospital taken over, but as the availability of these facilities could never be relied upon it still had to be completely self-sufficient. The expanding hospital marquee would always remain the basic unit of accommodation in which to care for the wounded and the sick.

The Corps was responsible also for such things as the control of water supplies, the prevention of epidemics, the supervision of hygiene and the protection of the army against tropical diseases. With its branch the Army Blood Transfusion Service, it had to collect and to supply thousands upon thousands of pints of blood and plasma, in conditions in which complete sterility was difficult to achieve, and to arrange the delivery of these essential transfusion fluids across hundreds of miles of desert or jungle track or battered roads, or to fly them close to the site of battle. When it is realised that blood can only be stored for at most some fourteen days and that never in the theatres of war in which I served after the defeat in France did we have anything but adequate amounts with which to transfuse our wounded, the efficiency with which this branch of the RAMC was organised can be appreciated.

Responsible for this service with the Middle East Forces and later with the British Liberation Army was the near genius Lieutenant-Colonel G. A. H. Buttle. A huge, kindly, chuckling bulk of a man, he was not only a doctor but also a scientist. Imperturbable, adored by his junior officers, he lit his organisation with such a flame of enthusiasm that no demand on the resources of the blood-transfusion service became too great or impossible to surmount. Send an urgent request to his headquarters from some forward unit and within hours the required blood would arrive, often brought in by one of his staff who would remain to help with the resuscitation of the wounded. And sometimes among the ice-containers of transfusion fluids would be packed a restorative bottle of Scotch. It was due to his unit and the services it provided that we as surgeons were sometimes able to achieve the seemingly impossible and return life to those who, without its help and dedication, would certainly have died.

No. 6 General Hospital was to be one of those which, for the whole of its service in the Middle East, was to be tented: a small town of sand-coloured marquees in the desert at the side of the Suez Canal. When I arrived at the hospital in Luton there were many familiar faces and new ones as well. The army laid down its criteria of age and fitness for those who were to serve in distant theatres of war and many of its original officers including its senior staff had been given home postings. We had as our senior technical officers – those in charge of the medical and surgical divisions – two first-class former civilian consultants whose brilliance, drive and personality had already brought them to the top of the medical profession. Their keenness and efficiency spread into all ranks of the hospital and the successful working of every department was assured.

Colonel Simpson Smith, so sadly destined to be killed at Tobruk while making a gallant attempt to escape after having been taken prisoner, inspired us with ideas as to how we could improve the treatment of the wounded and promote their subsequent comfort. He brought with him certain surgical instruments that he himself had designed, including a special suction apparatus, not included in our equipment, which was to prove invaluable in the treatment of abdominal injuries. As a surgeon he was in the front rank. As an officer he remained always a civilian in uniform. Brigadier or private, I do not believe rank made any difference to him. They were just two more 'chaps' to be liked and treated just the same. He tried very hard to be an expert in drill and formation marching because he considered it an obligation to ensure that from a purely military point of view the RAMC should be held in high esteem; but like most doctors he would never have done much credit to a parade. However, the Corps was not the loser because of that. For a few brief months they had the services of a brilliant and tireless surgeon. Many troops who were in the hospital at Tobruk in the dark days of the summer of 1942 will remember him with deep affection. They know that outside where the sand blows restlessly and ceaselessly, outside the simmering whitened walls of the town, side by side with some of those he tried so desperately to save, lies a great and compassionate friend.

All officers going overseas had to complete a short course in tropical medicine. As I had been in Dover I had not attended one and after a short stay with the hospital I was sent to Millbank to fulfil this requirement. London, as a result of the bombing raids, seemed always to be on fire somewhere and the skies blazed red at night, hoses curling in the streets. Everywhere I saw ambulances and fire engines and demolition squads tearing down walls about to topple, dragging away great beams and girders, digging for any trapped, maybe alive, bodies. Every night brought the intermittent, pulsating drone of enemy bombers overhead, masses packed into the Underground stations, searchlights probing the skies, the screeching pitch and fall of air-raid sirens and the reassuring single note of the all-clear. And yet life and love went on. Tired men and women streamed from the stations to their work, shops, often glass-littered, were open for business, buses ran, picking their way around closed streets.

In the evenings after our work was done I found my way through blacked-out streets to keep precious dates with a girl I had met. She was a nurse in the army, also awaiting posting overseas, and for a few brief days she, too, was in London. When planes were overhead and we rushed into doorways to cling together, it did not matter if somewhere bombs were falling or metal fragments of shrapnel were showering down about us like broken twigs in a great gale. With hell all around us, we were in heaven. And one morning I found red roses in a florist shop to send to her, red roses for remembrance. In the middle of the course, her embarkation orders came through. London became an even sadder place and my anguish was all-consuming, rather like the flames in the City and in the East End. I did not leave the officers' mess at night any more.

Our brief course ended. It had been brilliantly done because whatever deficiencies in certain specialities may have existed in the RAMC in peacetime, that of tropical medicine was not one. Its contribution to the subject had been great as a result of its decades of service and research into the medical problems of the tropical countries in which it largely served.

Before returning to Luton there were rushed visits to outfitters to buy items of hot-weather kit, including a completely and utterly useless topee. I wonder how many thousands of pounds of public money and how many thirty shillings of officers' savings were wasted on topis? In the climate of the Middle East they were never necessary and after having been dragged around they were eventually discarded with other unnecessary encumbrances. Still, money in wartime comes easily and goes with equal facility, so that tens of thousands of pounds of public expenditure or a few shillings of each officer's savings worries no one very unduly. But troops hate topis. They know they look quite at their worst in them and, strange as it may seem, the average soldier likes to look well dressed. What really makes him angry is when a routine order comes out enforcing the wearing of the hated headgear and at some inspection or other official function he sees the originator of this order parading in a service cap and looking cool and comfortable, relaxed and happy in the knowledge that he does not look like a Nervo and Knox Crazy Gang caricature of a soldier. Such hypocrisy the troops as well as the officers resent with remarkable thoroughness.

Although in my story I have not yet left Luton, my mind is carried forward to an occasion in Alexandria when we were due to change from summer to winter clothing. Even in that shining climate the weather can still play pranks and when it is due to turn cold it can surprise everyone by stacking on a belated spell of intense heat. Such an Indian summer irradiated this November and the date for our change of clothing was progressively postponed. But the weather must be subservient to brigadiers, and in spite of the heat it was so far past the time of year we were meant to change uniform that change we did. It was swelteringly hot on that first day of battledress. All we could hope was that the brigadier, far better covered than any of us, was dripping sweat a little faster than ourselves, even to the extent of being overcome by the heat. But in the midst of our evil hopes and to our disgust and bitter disillusionment a cool and relaxed brigadier walked into the hospital to see our commanding officer clothed in summer shorts and bush shirt!

I returned to No. 6 General Hospital to help with its final stages of preparation. Towards the end of that year of 1940 it seemed that a miracle had happened. Far away, where we were due to go, a small army was chasing a foe many times greater in number. Wavell had unleashed his few thousand troops and supported by the lightest of armour they were meeting with unbelievable success. Sollum fell. Bardia over the hill beyond Mussolini's outpost Fort Capuzzo gave way before the victorious advance, while prisoners in their thousands found their own way eastwards into the prisoner-of-war cages. It seemed to us, as it had seemed to our fathers in 1914 waiting impatiently at home, that all would be over in that theatre of war before we even arrived. The prospect that nearly three years of ding-dong struggle in the desert lay ahead, that attack after attack would peter out because of lack of supplies and difficulties of transport and communications, and weakness of direction, and would sometimes end in retreat, did not seem possible at that time. One was afraid of arriving too late – and yet there was to be time for the slowest sluggard.

While we waited, a night came when waves of bombers flew over on their way to Coventry, destined to introduce a new verb, 'to coventrate', meaning to destroy by mass bombing, into the English language. As for London, the Blitz had failed to bring the city to its knees and the cross on the dome of St Paul's, a symbol of survival, inspired the same hope another cross had inspired at a place called Calvary. But the resurrection of Europe lay far ahead.

And then came the order. In twenty-four hours we were to move. At the appointed hour we piled into the train in high spirits – until suddenly, as we drew slowly out of the station, the excitement of being underway evaporated. We had started, but we had parted too from all we knew, and an ache had begun to grow because there was nothing to sustain us in an uncertain future except memories which would have to be elastic enough to stretch over the coming years; in the stretching some of them broke.

6

VOYAGE TO SUEZ

NOVEMBER 1940–FEBRUARY 1941

Embarkation on Clydeside; voyage to Suez aboard the
Nea Hellas *with stopover in Durban*

At Yorkhill Quay in Glasgow, the dockside was lined with transports bearing names famous in ports throughout the world. Their vast outlines loomed through a gathering fog. Some still wore their peacetime colours and others had changed into the grey wartime utility suiting.

In the quayside sheds men were assembled for embarkation, waiting apathetically and patiently as soldiers are wont to do. Always there seemed to be delays, always the programme of any move allows hours of margin. It was a quiet crowd, thinking and wondering, and the only noise came from the derricks and cranes loading the equipment of war into the ships.

Side by side with us, due to embark on the same ship, the *Nea Hellas*, were Australian troops. They had journeyed thousands of miles but arrived too late to take part in the battle on the Continent, and now they were waiting to go back half the distance they had come. Fifteen months of trying to find a place to fight in, and now the prospect of another few months' search, was proving too much for the discipline of some of them. They had come to fight and so far there had not been any fighting for them, and they were 'browned off' to borrow from the soldiers' vocabulary. Eventually we embarked.

I think that many of us were dismayed by the difference between the accommodation provided for officers and that for other ranks, but how it could have been arranged otherwise in those early days of mass transport is difficult to see. As the war progressed and the ships were altered, more officers were accommodated in each cabin and provision for them approached the simplicity of other ranks. But in the early days there was too much difference and it led to considerable ill feeling. The average English soldier knows that he is going to have a difficult time with very little comfort, and with much grumbling and a considerable amount of colourful cursing, he accepts it in good humour. But our Australian comrades had a different outlook on life and considered, probably quite rightly, that what was good enough for an officer was good enough for them.

Down below, between decks, the troops marked out the little patch of ground that was to be theirs for two months. Later in the voyage, when the cold murk of English winter turned to the blaze of tropical summer, large air vents had to be installed in an endeavour to bring draughts of air into these stifling holds in which hundreds upon hundreds of men had their homes. On deck there was not enough space to sleep and so they were forced down below. Many of the ships of the convoy, including ours, were built for the stormy weather of the North Atlantic, not for voyaging in tropical seas, and with the still further lack of ventilation enforced by blackout regulations, at night the ship's company sweltered and sweated. Thousands of men were to travel like this, in gross discomfort. They were to travel as thousands of pilgrims travel from Singapore and Calcutta, from Penang and Bombay on their way to the port of Jeddah, gateway to the holy city of Mecca, herded together between decks. These soldiers, too, were pilgrims, following the god of war wherever he chose to set up his temple for worship and sacrifice.

We lay in Glasgow docks for a week, held up by a yellow, evil fog, and save for an occasional route march, confined to the ship. To our Australian comrades such an order was obviously attributable to sheer red tape and asking to be broken, and in spite of their own guards being at the gangway, they forced their way past to roam the city's taverns. But one day, when the sun broke through the pall of filth that hung above the city, the ship started on its voyage with all present and correct.

As we noses slowly down the Clyde, other great transports were edging out from the docks into the main stream, falling in line ahead to join this armada sailing to a war seven thousand miles away. The beautiful *Cape Town Castle*, glistening in the heliotrope, red and cream of happier times, was pushed out into the river, its deck rails crowded with troops strangely silent like those on all the ships. There were no false feelings of the glory and glamour of war. Most of those aboard wanted to go out to the Middle East and would have hated to be left behind because there at least was the prospect of action, not the monotonous routine of soldiering at home. But the loneliness and emptiness of parting brings hurt just the same.

Down the riverside, the air was loud with the noise of riveting. It was heartening to see these hundreds of ships being built, but a sad thought that it was only war that had brought this wave of prosperity to Britain's shipyards. A few years earlier, these yards were empty, the cranes and the slipways rusting from disuse, the craftsmen lounging in disillusioned idleness. Now not enough ships could be built.

We anchored off Greenoch where the huge convoy was assembling. In the distance, hills blue in the winter sunshine looked down on this silver stretch of water now filled with great liners and warships. The anchorage was full of activity with small boats hurrying between the transports on urgent last-minute business. One brought the news that one of the largest ships – a French liner – had broken down and would not be sailing, but from it a draft of officers was to be transferred to our ship. One of the doctors in this draft said that the conditions of overcrowding were so bad in the ship he had just left that he thought they would be bringing up their dead had they sailed into the tropics like that; men would be dying of heatstroke. He was glad that the ship's engines had failed.

Heatstroke is a problem that had to be faced and combated, especially in crowded ships sailing up the Red Sea in the heat of summer. It is a condition in which the heat-regulating mechanism of the body becomes overwhelmed by external conditions so that the temperature of the body steadily rises until it becomes life-threatening. Normally the temperature of the human body is maintained at an almost constant level, whatever the temperature of the surroundings. At the South Pole or in tropical Africa, whatever extremes the temperature reaches outside, the body is maintained at about 98 degrees Fahrenheit.

The control of temperature is delicate. Heat is lost in the main by the evaporation of sweat from the body surface and from the moisture in the lungs, and in order to provide blood and fluid to the sweat glands in the skin the superficial smaller arteries dilate. In cold weather the loss of heat is reduced to a minimum by the absence of sweating and the contraction of the arteries. The sweat glands and these arteries are under the automatic control of a heat-regulating centre in the brain. In response to minute rises in temperature of the blood supplying this centre, reflex nervous impulses at once cause dilatation of the arteries and increase sweating, thereby lowering the body temperature to normal. If, however, conditions are such that the air temperature is very high and the humidity of the atmosphere is great, the evaporation of sweat is lowered and the body temperature steadily rises until the individual is overwhelmed with the heat of his own body and may become delirious, pass into coma or even die.

Overcrowding lessens the circulation of air, makes it more humid and predisposes men to heatstroke in tropical conditions. These conditions were by the circumstances of war ever-present in the transports sailing in the tropics. The ships were for the most part not designed for hot-weather voyages, and medical officers were constantly on the watch for ominous signs. It says much for the improvised ventilation that ship's companies contrived that cases were few, but to overcrowd beyond a maximum could court disaster.

One grey morning, when the winter sun had given way to overcast skies and rain, we sailed away. In the lightening day, the Mull of Kintyre and the north coast of Ireland were silhouetted against the morning sky. For miles over the cold sea the convoy stretched, guarded by toy-like destroyers on the horizon of each flank and by the grey bulk of a battleship ploughing its way through choppy waves. Day after day we were to see the same ships in the same positions, as though they had been tied to each other by cables. Each morning you could go on deck and see your friend the *Franconia* or cross to the opposite side and see the *Duchess of Bedford*, affectionately known as the 'Drunken Duchess'. Only on some nights could you see the dim outlines of your neighbours, but you knew they were there, going onward, onward, relentlessly, interminably. We would go west first, beating out of the range of enemy aircraft, then we would veer southwest and finally south, but all the time the convoy kept to its unchangeable pattern until it seemed that we were standing still and that it was the sea and the sky, bringing with them the warmth and the sunshine, that were rushing past us.

Days merged into one another, as they would on a peacetime voyage, until they become lost in their sameness. On the limited deck space we had daily parades, competitions and lectures but there was still plenty of time to idle by in the increasing heat. Sometimes we played deck quoits or shuffleboard but even these monotony-relieving games the troops could not play because the deck space was so limited. But it was at night, when the ship was almost battened down in its blackout and the men were herded below in half-lit between decks, dripping with sweat, that conditions were at their worst. There was nothing we could do about it; there was not enough room for them all to sleep on deck.

It was perhaps small wonder that troops on these long voyages, in conditions that to say the least were hard, had many matters about which to complain, especially as they had such long, empty hours on their hands. In so far as was possible, the welfare officer of the ship and the unit officers did their best with concerts, boxing matches and the like; of all the sports the boxing was the most popular. In the heavier weights the RAMC could not compete on very even terms with our far larger rivals, but in the lighter weights it was a different story. Their bodies may have looked less tanned by the sun, they may have lived in streets where smoke-laden air filtered away all health-giving rays, but for all this in enthusiasm, spirit and skill they were more than a match for their Australian friends. All of the ship's company who were not on duty turned out to see these fights. Clinging to masts, scrambling on the air vents, onlookers sought every possible vantage point, ready to cheer victor and vanquished, generous in their praise for any worthy fighter whether he came from the wide spaces of Down Under or from the closely crowded streets of Glasgow.

For a while everything was forgotten save this sport. Across the water separating the ships, equally crowded mastheads could be seen where also the war, with all its uncertainties, its heartaches and its worries, was being forgotten in a few hours of vigorous fun. I think that as a result of these boxing matches, our Australian shipmates looked with added respect on the RAMC. Perhaps after all they were not just a bunch of weaklings who had joined or been posted to the medical corps because they were not fit for any good fighting battalion. Perhaps after all they were just as much a part of this great army as they themselves.

Food was always a subject about which there was much grumbling, sometimes justifiable, sometimes serving as an outlet for other pent-up feelings. One day, two Australians presented themselves before the duty medical officer wearing their gas masks and holding before them two plates of fish. The complaint was that the fish smelt so high that it was quite inedible. Now a complaint offered in such a way in the British Army would be unlikely to reach an officer and would be dealt with along comparatively severe lines. It would be held as conduct prejudicial to good order and discipline, a section of King's Regulations that covers a multitude of sins. But armies vary and certainly in the Australian battalion on our ship this was regarded as a very justifiable means of offering a complaint. If there was to be a complaint, why should it not be clothed in a certain amount of reasonable humour? The medical officer concerned was a wise man, he did not stand on a pillar of unnecessary dignity and take disciplinary action, but he asked one of the men to get a knife and fork. He then proceeded to eat both plates of fish and afterwards remarked that the men could remove their respirators as the cause of the bother had been eradicated. Although he did not enjoy the fish, it was not as bad as all that.

We were living side by side with men whose ideas were not the same as ours. Their lives at home were freer, with fewer grades of society than existed in England. Our sense of discipline was very different, but in the weeks that we were herded together we learnt to like and respect each other in spite of all the differences. Sometimes we could not agree with their ideas, but if they were going to fight as bravely and as gallantly as their fathers had done before them, these differences did not really matter. We all belonged to the British Commonwealth of Nations, we spoke the same language, we had the same sovereign king, but these links that bound us did not necessarily have to mean we were nations with the same characteristics. If we were to succeed in friendliness and alliance, we had to recognise and respect our differences.

Jan. 23 No. 64 General Hospital, MEF, GHQ, 2nd Echelon

My dear Mum and Dad,
This convoy is very interesting, but of course I can tell you nothing about it. In fact there is very little I can say that the censor would like.

We are now getting nicely hot. We are in tropical uniform and most of us are looking like boiled lobsters. It seems extraordinary to think of an English winter here as we bask in this hot sunshine. We still do quite a lot of work as we have a far too military minded Lt.Col who thinks we should all know how to about turn and salute and all that sort of nonsense like the brigade of guards. But perhaps he'll get tired before we do. Anyhow, the Australians on board say they'll chuck him overboard for £10 so we might have to get up a subscription...

At night the blackout makes everywhere very hot as we can't have any windows open at all and I've no doubt it will be very much worse later on as it will be summer time south of the line.

The flying fishes are beginning to make their appearance once again and it is all rather reminiscent of the old Antilochus days [a reference to my father's days as a ship's surgeon 1937–8] though very different in circumstances.

We all get on very well with the Aussies although they are a very tough crowd. I'm very pleased I'm not an Italian because I'm quite sure there's a hell let loose when they have the good fortune to meet them.

Well I think that's all I can tell you at the minute.

My love to you both.

★   ★   ★

About two and a half weeks out from England the convoy changed its direction and broke formation as we neared Freetown and the ships sailed into the port. For mile upon mile the single line of transports stretched, still guarded by its naval escort, although the battleship protection had left us near Gibraltar.

Can anyone fail to be thrilled by the sight of a new continent about which they have imagined so much? Ahead lay the ghastliness and horror of a war; far behind was a place of belonging and of golden memories, unforgettable and always living; but in between was this land of mystery and romance. We stood and gazed at blue hills covered in a shimmering mist and sparkling yellow sands lapped by turquoise seas and surrounded by an arc of still palms. In the protection of the harbour the heat beat down from the heavens until the metal rungs of the ship were like fire to touch. We were on the fringe of an exotic world which most of us had never seen before, and we were on our way to live for years in other fabled lands.

The ship sailed into a vast natural harbour, but anchored way out from the shore in an endeavour to be out of the flying range of the malaria-carrying mosquito. These insects normally have a comparatively short range of flight, and only when carried on a wind do they travel miles from their breeding grounds. Armies in the past have been decimated and rendered useless as fighting forces by the ravages of malaria, and it speaks highly for all branches of the RAMC that by its methods to combat this disease, although cases were inevitable, it has avoided epidemics.

Hardly had each ship anchored at its berth before it was surrounded by small native boats, whose occupants were ready to trade their mangoes, bananas, oranges and other local fruits or any of their tribal trinkets in exchange for anything they could get. These 'bumboats', with Bible texts often written on one side and blasphemy on the other, did a roaring trade in spite of every order that had been issued forbidding the buying of fruit from these natives. Although there is an undoubted risk of the spread of infective fevers such as typhoid and dysentery from eating untreated fruit, it was in a way a foolish order if it was to be given without the power to enforce it. In any case, as soon as the troops landed at a port, fruit, which had been very scarce during the voyage, would be one of their earliest purchases and the risk was the same anywhere in countries where such diseases are endemic.

Owing to the mass immunisation of all troops against fevers of the typhoid type, the incidence of such disease was very small throughout the campaign in the Middle East. And as one seemed as likely to get dysentery in the middle of the desert living on army rations as from eating fruit in Alexandria or Cairo, the infection being so often flyborne, the added risk to the troops from the bumboats was small. Apart from the fruit itself, the long bargaining was a source of constant delight and amusement to troops likely to become bored with the convoy's delay, but many must have been short of blankets and shirts and pants as a result of the exchanges that went on. Sometimes the bartering, often interrupted by streams of water from the ships hoses as attempts were made to drive the bumboats off, was over small monkeys which, wide-eyed and terrified, would be hauled up the side of the ship in baskets for inspection by prospective buyers. The ever-ready cockney wit rapidly asserted itself, with cries of, 'How many blankets do you want for an elephant?'

One day while we lay anchored in the harbour, bursts of ack-ack fire from every ship suddenly disturbed the peace as an enemy observation aircraft came over to check up on the shipping. It was apparently a regular visitor and sadly bore the markings of Vichy France. It was a shame that some of those who had fought side by side with our armies in the disaster of the battle of France had forgotten comradeships and loyalties and had joined our enemies. When we left Freetown a few days later we passed the wreckage of what had once been a ship, floating and bobbing in an oily sea. Perhaps this was the victim of such a reconnoitring aircraft, which had betrayed it to waiting raiders and submarines. Fortunately those who were against us in France were in the small minority. For the vast number, all hope, however secret it was, rested on Britain. Hate for the enemy smouldered on.

As soon as the convoy had watered and fuelled, once again, one by one, the ships sailed out and onwards towards the south, resuming formation like a well-trained company of troops as soon as the open sea was reached. The next stop was Cape Town or Durban and the ship's company settled down to passing the time in lectures, interminable deck sports, the preparation for the inevitable ceremony of crossing the line, and hour upon hour of getting browner and more accustomed to the increasingly fierce tropical sun.

Periodically we had boat drill – but we never knew whether

it was real or not. the early dawn of one morning the alarm bells sounded. The quartermaster of a medical unit rose drowsily from his bed and with muttered oaths he seized his life jacket and looked around for his cap, which he could not find. In desperation he grasped his topee and rushed up on deck. In his pyjamas and his life jacket with the topee upon his head he stood there uncomfortably, wondering what on earth he looked like dressed in such an odd garb. Most of his fellows were hatless or wearing the ordinary service cap. It soon became obvious that this was a practice and the inspecting party came around the ship's deck. To his intense surprise, the quartermaster was picked upon. 'The only sensible man on the ship,' said the inspecting officer. 'Here is a man who is wise enough to know that if he is going to spend a number of days in an open boat in this climate, he will need some protection.'

It had seemed likely from the first day we boarded the ship that the voyage was not going to be easy. If combatant troops in the midst of war could treat an order forbidding them to go ashore with disdain and receive no punishment for this disregard, it didn't augur well for the ensuing months. This Australian division was equally divided between our ship and the SS *Franconia* and on each was the personnel of a large general hospital, including nurses and associated medical units. The division contained a small number of very tough characters and unhappily it was these, and not the vast majority of their fellow soldiers, who made the voyage a difficult one.

It was obviously right to scatter units of various regiments so that in the event of the loss of a ship at least part of any formation would survive, but it was unwise to include non-combatant troops with those of another country unless discipline was strict. It was an error to mix soldiers who were forbidden to gamble with those among whom were many whose main occupation, night and day, was playing cards in a 'two up' school where money changed hands; or to join together in cramped quarters those who were accustomed to treating their officers with a certain respect with others who, as often as not, familiarly called their commanding officer 'Bert'. I think that had this Australian division sailed with a fighting unit of the British Army, with its tradition of discipline, trouble would have been avoided.

As it was, orders prohibiting smoking on deck after dark lest the striking of a match endanger the whole convoy were frequently ignored. The lifeboat covers were slashed and their emergency supplies removed. As the ship sailed into the hot weather the indiscipline seemed to grow worse. Somewhere below the lower decks the ship's store of liquor lay. A very extensive operation involving the removal of the intervening decking was undertaken to uncover this and it was some time before the cause of the resulting drunkenness was traced to this audacious break-in

Each night a round of inspection was supposed to be carried out by a patrol headed by an officer of the RAMC or of the Australian division, but as the weeks went by it became increasingly apparent that our counterparts were very averse to carrying out these duties when things were rough down below and they were often performed by the sergeant alone. After we left Freetown there were vague rumours that a steward on the ship carrying the other part of this division, who had failed to cooperate in the supply of beer, had disappeared overboard. The rumour may have been false, but it was one that caused disquiet amongst certain officers.

A friend of mine, the pathologist attached to our hospital, was one day leaning over the rails watching the flying fish. An Australian came up the hatchway on to the officers' deck. 'Have you got a light?' he said. 'I don't smoke,' replied the major. 'You wouldn't, you fucking English pommy bastard,' was the Aussie's comment. Major Post, the officer concerned, had boxed for his university and his reaction was to hit the soldier, who disappeared backwards down the hatchway and then picked himself up and stumbled away. The major was immediately conscious of the enormity of his offence – striking a soldier. He had visions of court martials and of being dismissed from the service. He awaited the course of events that might follow anxiously, but the next day the soldier with his black eye approached him and said, 'I deserved that punch and I'd like to apologise for what I said. Can we shake hands?' They did and the matter was ended.

On one occasion an RAMC sergeant was detailed to assemble a fatigue party. He had gathered together three out of the four required and on seeing someone leaning over the side tapped him on the shoulder and said, 'What are you doing?' The soldier turned round and proved to be one of the rather difficult Australians. 'I'm minding my own fucking business. What are you doing?' The sergeant thought that discretion was the better part of valour and looked elsewhere for the fourth member of his party.

As we neared Cape Town, the news went around that half the convoy was going to put into this port and the rest, including our ship, was to proceed to Durban. The Australians had visited Cape Town on their voyage to England where they had been royally entertained and where the daughters had not all been locked up. There was, naturally, bitter disappointment that this old acquaintance was not to be renewed, and one night all possible water taps were turned on in an endeavour to force the *Nea Hellas* into Cape Town. Water was very scarce in the last few days before reaching Durban and all officers were summoned to be addressed by the ship's captain. His name I believe was Captain Burn, senior in the line and the author of several books. His message to us was succinct and acerbic. He said that he had been carrying troops throughout the last war and during this, and that he had been proud of every voyage he had made. On this occasion he was ashamed of the ship, ashamed of the troops and in particular of the officers, who were supposed to have maintained discipline. He walked out in fury.

All of us who visited Durban will remember not only the loveliness of the town, with its fine waterfront edged by high white buildings and hotels, but also the welcome we received from the population. It was not a haphazard welcome, but an organised one and none the less sincere for that. We were taken to silver sands lapped in cobalt by the sea, where we bathed and lazed. We were entertained at lunches and dinners and driven out to the hills to visit native kraals (villages) – all of us, officers, NCOs, nurses and men. Our hosts were kind enough to allow us time to ourselves and some of us wandered round the town or took rickshaws pulled by Zulus wearing feathered headgear. We did not know that because of the strenuous work their job entailed, their lifespan was reduced by decades. We were in an unreal world, a halfway house between war and peace. We clung tightly to life and love because in the end life was love.

Each evening we returned to our ship and late on each of these nights the military police from the town unloaded their Commonwealth cargoes on to the quayside. Some moved and some were so still they seemed to be dead. They were carried up the gangway and down below decks to recover by the morrow.

We left Durban, and the buildings and hotels on the waterfront grew gradually smaller and more indistinct. Many must have wondered whether to make their lives in this seemingly lovely country when the war had ended. As it was, we sailed a hundred and nine short of our full complement. To our relief, mustering all the personnel of the medical units, we found our strength intact. Perhaps at least some of those stragglers caught a later boat to join the armies in the desert? Was it due to this loss that our journey towards and through the Red Sea, in spite of the increasing heat, proved almost uneventful? Only one incident stood out and this I have to recount as, indirectly, it was to affect my future postings in the RAMC.

I was duty medical officer when an Australian attended the sick parade. He had a grossly swollen right hand due to a fractured bone. He said that while he had been sleeping on deck because in the heat he had found sleep impossible below, an attempt had been made to bugger him. He had leapt up, recognised in the moonlight an officer in the RAMC, although he was only dressed in pyjamas, and promptly hit him; in so doing he had broken his hand. He wished that a charge be brought against his assailant. I dealt with his broken bone and handed over the conduct of the other affair to the company officer. An enquiry was instituted and it was decided that the officer concerned should appear before a court martial on arrival in Egypt. I thought that for me this was the end of the matter, but when we finally arrived at a transit camp in the desert, No. 6 General Hospital was ordered to prepare for service in Greece. To my dismay and astonishment I was removed from the strength of the hospital so that I could be in the country at the time of the court martial and was posted to Cairo merely to give evidence to the effect that the injury for which I had treated the Australian was compatible with hitting someone very hard with a closed fist. Divisions, with their Greek allies, were fighting to hold the German-reinforced Italian army across the Mediterranean, but justice apparently had to be done, and seen to be done, although men were dying by the score on the Greek archipelago.

Back on the ship, we had yet to arrive in Egypt. Sailing north, we separated from a part of the convoy bound for East Africa but were joined, cheeringly, by two French ships flying the flag of Free France. Not all had listened to Pétain, 'the old man of Vichy'. Finally, we arrived at Port Taufiq, near Suez. The port was packed with transports and merchant ships of every description, each awaiting their turn to discharge. Every berth was filled. Tanks, guns, lorries and stores lined the quayside and hundreds upon hundreds of troops filed down the gangways. So full was the port that we had to wait nearly two days before there was room for us to tie up, and then the Australians were the first to disembark. It had been a voyage made difficult by the few and not by the majority – who were all fine men – and most of the former we had left behind in Durban. But there was no doubt that discipline had not stood the strain of nearly eighteen months of inaction and the division was probably to suffer for this with unnecessary casualties in the battles that lay ahead. We waved them goodbye. In a few weeks' time they were to be fighting and dying in Greece and Crete and I was to see some of them once again, lying wounded in wards of No. 64 General Hospital in Alexandria.

7

LANDING AT SUEZ

FEBRUARY–MARCH 1941

*The vast encampment at El Quassasin;
the first of many visits to Cairo*

Even on this early-spring day the sun shone hotly and our eyes
were dazzled by the light bouncing off the whitened
buildings as we left the ship and paraded with our equipment on
the dockside. From Suez we travelled by train to the Canal Zone
where many of the large hospitals were being established and where
the main bases for the army were already set up. As the train drew
slowly through the town, crowds of children and beggars lined the
railroad, clamouring and shouting with outstretched arms, and they
reaped a rich reward. The British soldier is famous for the soft spot
he has in his heart for children and he was not yet conversant with
the wiles of these urchins. Moreover, he was not yet accustomed
to the constant demand for *baksheesh*, which, if ever responded to,
produced in a twinkling a crowd of clutching hands and screaming

voices as if from nowhere. He was new on the scene and responded to the apparent welcome with sweets, food, cigarettes and small coins. However, he was not slow to learn, and in a very few weeks became almost allergic to the sight of any small boy, and with a few quickly learned Egyptian oaths and a sprinkling of his customary vocabulary would send him smartly on his way. The inhabitants of Suez must have blessed the fact that they were so situated that they only had to deal with novices who seldom returned.

The train ran northwards through the cultivated delta where every inch of space was made to grow its thrice-yearly crop. Artificial irrigation by canals of water draining from the Nile into innumerable smaller channels had brought prosperous farming to the mudflats stretching on either side of the great river, at least to the owners of the land. From the channels the water was raised to the fields by primitive devices: by buckets using the most elementary system of levers, by the Archimedes' screw invented more than two hundred years before the birth of Christ, and sometimes by blindfolded bullocks pursuing their never-ending circle harnessed to a radial beam. The grain was separated from the chaff by the wind, and the wheat ground into flour by ageless stones that might have been used when Thebes and Luxor were important cities in the ancient world. Scattered throughout the delta were villages, poverty-stricken collections of huts built of mud and straw and dung baked hard in the blazing sun, where animals and humans shared the same roof as they had in medieval England. The fellahin leave these villages with the first light of dawn, and only when the last of the sun is fading from the sky is the journey home begun. If the worker is the lucky possessor of an ass it is he who usually rides while his wife plods steadily behind, a heavy load supported on her head; but sometimes both mount the unhappy animal.

We disembarked from our train at El Quassasin, a small village halt a few miles from the cultivated area. In the sand around were the tented homes of thousands of British troops. We were still rookies at the art of living in Egypt but the experience of one of our lieutenant-colonels taught us a lot. He had taken off his pack and webbing while we were awaiting lorries to transport us to our section of the camp. In the half-dark a crowd of apparently friendly children gathered round him chattering away and all smiles. One minute they seemed to be there and the next the small crowd had simply dissolved and all that could be seen were flying figures in the gathering dusk, but the colonel's pack was flying with them, never to be seen again.

On arrival at a transit camp in this desert town we learned that we were not to set up there but to await transport for Alexandria and thence for Greece. In point of fact the unit never sailed, although all the heavy baggage was embarked, as by that time it was obvious that retreat from our last foothold in Europe was inevitable.

It was an amazing camp, this at El Quassasin. Hundreds of tents stretched in all directions for miles on end. Roads had been constructed through the sand, water towers and water pipes laid down, baths and latrines erected in this wilderness. The NAAFI, occupying a small village of tents of its own, was there and already open-air cinemas were making their appearance. A population equivalent to that of a medium-sized town was living in this waste of sand.

Large hospitals, to accommodate two thousand patients each, had already arrived and one with its pathological laboratories, X-ray units and operating theatres was already busy. Most of the accommodation was in the large expanding type of marquee, although as these hospitals were destined for permanent use during the campaign, the operating theatres were constructed of local light mud and bricks.

One of the great difficulties in carrying out surgery in sand areas is the presence of dust. The slightest wind will raise clouds, which will percolate into an operating theatre unless the building is made proof against it. It is quite impossible to proof a tent and as the dust may carry with it germs which will infect the exposed wounds during an operation, its exclusion is desirable if possible. Naturally in the forward units such perfection was impossible, but in the static base units everything was done to reduce this added risk.

All the marquees were dug in, that is to say the floor was excavated to a depth of about three feet so that the beds were all below the surface level. Thus in the event of air attack the patient was protected from blast and flying metal fragments. This digging in had the advantage of giving more space in each marquee. Already English ingenuity was persuading flowers to spring from barren sand, and paths and stonework lent relief to its interminable sameness.

Here then, hospital units were setting up, offering to their patients diagnosis and treatment and nursing as skilled and as efficient as that which the civilian could obtain in any of the major cities in England. In this sandy waste were clean sheets and beds. Far from home, sick or wounded, the soldier was learning that he would be cared for by the RAMC and the Queen Alexandra nurses as well as was humanly possible, no matter where he found himself.

A little outside this base complex were barbed-wire-protected pens into which the prisoners of war from the desert campaign were herded until they could be sorted out, interrogated and finally sent to permanent camps. There were those occupied by the Italians and others in which the Libyan levies, Mussolini's empire army, were confined, and in both we helped with the many sick parades which were required for these thousands of men. Some of the native troops were but boys of twelve or thirteen. To recruit these levies the Italians had ordered each headman of a village to provide a certain number of conscripts, and as he had no wish to lose most of his adult men, lads were sent to make up the numbers. All were delighted to be prisoners and out of a war they did not understand and in which they had no wish to engage. Some two thousand of them had apparently deserted during the campaign and had gone over en masse to the British lines waving pieces of white material. The officer who was to have accepted their surrender told them that he was too busy to cope with them, but if they liked to come back on the following day he would see what he could do. They disappeared into the desert and returned happily the following day.

This enormous camp was a happy hunting ground for the crowds of local Egyptians. Many were employed in the various labour duties that accompanied the construction and maintenance of this vast base. Many others were there to see what they could get. Not since the golden days of the 1914–18 War had there been such Allah-sent opportunities for fleecing the infidel. It would have been a breach of faith had the occasion not been seized upon and fully developed. They were a green lot, these soldiers. They did not know the difference between a good piastre coin and a very poorly counterfeited one. They had not the slightest idea of the value of a fly whisk or a leather-covered piece of wood, and if they left unguarded valuable personal belongings in their tents or stacked piles of blankets and sheets or tins of petrol and oil, perhaps protected only by a little barbed wire, well praise be again to Allah.

The canvas from the tents was much sought after and a few seconds' work with a sharp knife would lead to the reward of a large panel from one of the sidewalls. A whole tent might be the prize, spirited away in the growing dusk, especially when a unit was out on manoeuvres and perforce an inadequate number of guards had been left behind. There was an occasion when a well-known Harley Street surgeon and his tent mate retired to bed one night only to wake next morning and find that all their personal belongings and clothing, as well as the side walls of their small marquee, had disappeared. The language of a doctor on such an occasion, miles away from the restraining influence of that dignified street, is well up into the bargee class, especially when it is aggravated by the unsympathetic merriment of his colleagues.

The energetic pilfering spread all over Egypt as the months went by. At first it was easy, but even when it was less so it still went on. Lorries and army cars would disappear from closely guarded parks. To leave a car unattended for a few minutes was to invite disaster; if the car itself remained on one's return something was sure to have gone – the spare wheel, the radiator cap, a petrol can – and if the delay was lengthy it was not exceptional to find the vehicle jacked up on bricks with the wheels removed. Periodically, dumps of stolen army stores would be recovered, but in spite of all the thefts continued. From a hospital in Alexandria one night, bales containing seven hundred blankets and a consignment of pyjamas vanished. Now and then a railway truck would fail to arrive and would be discovered some days later relieved of its contents.

In spite of knowing full well that petty as well as organised thieving was part of life among a considerable section of the community, some time or other you would be caught off your guard and some personal possession would disappear. Not an uncommon trick, and one that paid reasonable dividends, was for a newspaper boy to stick a paper under your nose inviting you to buy. Sometimes the paper was a current issue, occasionally it was not, but the few brief moments during which the *Egyptian Mail* had been pushed into your face had been time enough for the small boy's accomplice to extract a wallet or fountain pen that may have been inadvertently showing above the flap of your pocket. The loss, of course, you would not discover for a while and then it was too late. Had you in addition purchased the paper, the whole operation would quite obviously have been an unqualified success.

Much of the minor thieving that went on was engendered by gross poverty, the poverty that reduced a man to borderline destitution, so that nothing mattered provided the bare necessities of life could be bought and, very occasionally, a luxury obtained. It was not money that was the root of all evil, but poverty. Had it been possible to earn a wage, small by European standards but a wage that banished the fear and worry of want, reasonable honesty would have replaced dishonesty.

Outstanding in their quality of impeccable honesty were the Sudanese, who in Cairo and Alexandria provided the finest type of servant. These men would come up from the Sudan and spend from three to four years in Egypt, during which time they would save enough money to be able to go home for six to nine months on holiday. When that money was spent they returned once again. They were fine men, often of imposing physique and proud in the knowledge that they were good at their job. Call them by error Egyptians and they were bitterly offended. In the eighteen months during which I was at No. 64 General Hospital in Alexandria, although we left personal possessions scattered about our rooms, never did we suffer the smallest theft when our servant staff was Sudanese.

★ ★ ★

As we were due to go to Greece in a very short time, we were given forty-eight hours' leave to visit Cairo. This was to be our one fleeting taste of a Near Eastern city before once again we went back to Europe; none of us dreamt that on and off for nearly three more years we would visit this capital. Cairo was to become the leave Mecca of the armies of the desert. In the sands, hot and dusty or bitterly cold and wet, the prospect of a brief trip to Cairo was always exciting. It meant a return to civilisation, a return to hot baths and clean clothes, to first-class food and drink and to the charm and pleasure of the company of women. Troops wanted to forget the war, to get away from all the discomfort and danger of their lives, and to Cairo they flocked.

One of the disadvantages of service outside Europe in the early years of the war was the fact that there were not enough suitable female companions for men on leave. The European population of any of these countries was very small compared with the number of soldiers who were spending their few precious days off in these cities. All the food and drink, all the cinemas, the shops, the hot baths and clean sheets did not compensate for the tenderness and comfort of having a girl companion with whom to go around. Troops saw only their fellow soldiers for month after month, and for a few brief days they wished, very naturally, to try and return to normal social life.

It was a problem to which the army and its welfare branches were very alive, and with the posting of women's services abroad and the provision of absolutely first-class clubs, steps were being made towards making that brief leave as happy as possible. After all, a happy leave meant a soldier with a higher morale. Perhaps from these friendships broken hearts and broken marriages sometimes resulted; on the other hand there were those that developed into deeply loving and understanding relationships. But for the most they were light and airy flirtations, enchanting just for the few days they survived, so that they ended only with happy memories that were taken back to the emptiness of the desert.

Any solutions, however, were only partial. Nothing would prevent the very natural urge of men to seek out women, especially among those men who had come down on leave from the desert battles where life in a second could be turned to death. Cairo and Alexandria abounded with prostitutes and the problem of venereal disease was a challenging one. The only certain way to avoid it was by the maintenance of continence based on a moral code of Christian belief. Inevitably, there were thousands who were not prepared to take that path. The welfare services, the church and all medical officers combined in their efforts to combat the risks, although the viewpoints from which the doctor and the padre approached the issue were very different.

Knowledge of the manifestations and dangers of the disease was disastrously lacking among the population from which the soldier was drawn. It was therefore one of the duties of all doctors in the Medical Corps, including its surgeons, to lecture on the serious problems to which both syphilis and gonorrhoea could give rise, and by engendering a very real fear of the possible consequences of infection, without exaggerating them in any way, to try and deter the soldier from risking his future health. Such lectures had been given to all troops on the ship during its voyage to the Middle East. When the average soldier understood that months of treatment could be his lot before he was finally cured – and these were the days before penicillin – he was apt to weigh in his mind whether the risk was worthwhile. It would have been unrealistic to believe that by education alone venereal disease would be eliminated from the forces, and inspected brothels, both for officers and men, were made available. The one for the former at Alexandria was known as 'Mary's' and it was almost in the nature of a club, with a bar where you could chat to a girl without any persuasion being exercised or any pressure to buy. During one of the raids on Alexandria, Mary's suffered a direct hit and there were numerous casualties, but it soon opened its doors again. Such centres were repugnant to the padres. They represented the failure of an ideal. Probably that was so, but where the ideology was rejected, practical methods had to come to the fore to maintain the health of fighting units. It was certainly true that as a result of the combined efforts of welfare officers, doctors and padres the incidence of the disease was very low. Ideals and practical methods together brought about these good results.

Cairo was a city of contrasts in which, since the time of

Napoleon, Western attitudes and methods had tried to usurp the ancient traditions and mode of living of the past, but they had not succeeded – and probably never will now that Egypt is more than ever pushing away its Western influences. You arrived at Cairo station; there you could choose either a broken-down taxi or a rickety horse-drawn carriage to drive you to your hotel. On your way to Shepheard's you passed the camel, with yellowed teeth, plodding its way sullenly through the capital, carrying its burden who knew where, or else the ass trotting jerkily along with its owner perched precariously (or so it seemed) well over the after end of the animal. But also you saw gigantic limousines, gleaming in the bright sunshine, each with the modern counterpart of some ancient potentate reclining prosperously in the back. It was natural enough to assume that these must be English merchants and traders who had lived in Egypt, extracting everything and giving nothing in return and owing a debt of gratitude to that country for all that it had done for them. At least it would be a pardonable error, based on an impression that many a good Egyptian would give us, but as you learned better you found that they were anything but English. Greek, French, Italian, Egyptian, American, but rarely English. The small and ancient car chugging along was his birthright and inheritance. For whatever faults he may have had, the average Englishman working in a country abroad felt that in him honest and fair dealing was on trial and he was determined that it should not be brought into low repute, even though the opportunity of attaining great wealth would have to be turned aside.

At Shepheard's you could enjoy every comfort offered by any of the great hotels of the cities of the world. You could sit out on the verandah, watching a colourful world pass by on the pavements before you, Western and Eastern intermingling but never mixing. A few yards away from this almost romantic hotel, you could lose yourself in streets that had been unchanged for hundreds of years, streets where the ways of the West were as alien then as they had ever been.

In the shops there was every luxury of modern life. Clothes woven by the finest English weavers, dresses designed by Parisian couturiers, jewellery, silver and gold, the work of the master craftsmen of the Western countries. Not far away, in the narrow shaded streets of the old bazaar, clothes, cloths, silver and gold work, all in abundant supply, but they were made by the same artisan methods that had produced similar merchandise hundreds of years gone by. Here in front of the visitor, the handloom still slowly wove exquisite patterns; here, where the smell of oriental spices and perfumes mixed in the still, hot air, the silversmith and goldsmith hammered their metal into intricate and delicate designs. Time stood still in this part of Cairo; whether English, Egyptians, Germans or Italians lived in the citadel dominating the city, it would not matter to the workers here. There would still be clients to buy their wares. As long as they were there, what did it matter where they came from, or whether they wore khaki or field grey, whether they spoke English or German?

To this city then, thousands upon thousands of troops looked for an escape from the tyranny of war and sand. They arrived dirty, dusty – yes, and smelly too – from the desert life and emerged from their hotels clean and smart and ready to enjoy their few days of liberty. They visited the mosques of which there are hundreds in the city, went out to the Pyramids, were photographed riding on camels or against the backdrop of the Sphinx. They were fleeced by a thousand rogues, mistakenly bought the artificial rather than the genuine, paid exorbitant prices for the presents they sent home, gave double or treble the legal taxi or cab fare, but it mattered little. They spent nothing for months on end in the desert and the strangeness and unreality and forgetfulness of their brief leave was worth it all.

In the evenings there were bars and dance halls and women, open-air cinemas and theatres and army clubs. There were lights in the city at night-time too, although there was a partial blackout, but to eyes accustomed to the deep darkness of the British version they appeared as bright and attractive as the neon lights of Piccadilly.

Memory is kind. Looking back on those periods of leave in Cairo one forgets the dust, the heat and the flies, the poverty and dirt and the beggars who thronged the streets. One forgets the crowds of small boys who pestered to be allowed to clean one's shoes, which before they threw filth on them had been sparkling in the sunshine. The dirty pictures surreptitiously extracted from the flowing robes of most street vendors, the invitations to meet 'my virgin sister', all this, real and ugly at the time though it was, lies deep in the background. Memory brings to the fore times of great happiness that still live vividly in the mind. It was the war that brought them about and when it ended, perhaps these recollections should have faded, but instead they refuse to be forgotten.

8

A COURT MARTIAL AND SUBSEQUENT POSTING

APRIL–MAY 1941

From the witness box in Cairo to duties at
No. 64 General Hospital in Alexandria

We arrived back at our camp to learn that things were going badly for the Western Desert Force. A well-disciplined and well-equipped division of the German army, trained under conditions simulating desert warfare, had been shipped across the Mediterranean. It was no longer a horde of ill-disciplined Italian troops and native levies that the small army of the Nile was up against, but a determined and deadly foe. The numbers of our own army had been depleted by the tragic need of Greece for support and help, and against this new enemy it slowly and steadily had to give ground. This enforced retreat left the German army masters of Benghazi and Derna. Short-circuiting Tobruk, whose garrison became enveloped and surrounded in one of the longest and most difficult sieges in history, their advance was halted only just short of the Egyptian frontier.

Across the sea the news was equally bad. Against Italian forces strongly reinforced by their German allies, British and Dominion troops with their Greek friends were fighting a rearguard action as they retreated towards the sea and evacuation. A heroic gesture of help and good faith was being beaten back by a superiority of arms and planes. But we had kept faith even though that meant a worsening of our own position in the desert, and perhaps in the long run, in view of the uncertain years of post-war instability, that gesture of good faith may have helped to bring peace to a world saddened and torn by mistrust.

Because No. 6 General Hospital's orders to proceed to Alexandria for embarkation to Greece had not yet been rescinded, and because I was to be a medical witness at the court martial of the officer who had been accused on the voyage to Egypt, I was removed from the strength of this unit and told to report to Cairo and to act as prisoner's escort. This was not a happy duty. An accused officer was forbidden to wear a Sam Browne belt (the belt supported by a narrow strap worn diagonally across the shoulder) so that it would be apparent to all wherever he appeared that he was under arrest. This was particularly important on the train and on entering or leaving the mess of the transit unit to which we were sent. The convening of the court martial in Cairo was to take several days, however. I therefore came to an understanding with my prisoner. We would leave the mess, he without his Sam Browne, which I had in a haversack. We would then proceed to the nearest hotel where I would give him the haversack and in the lavatory he would put on the belt. Both of us then left and went our own ways in Cairo, he having given me his word to meet me at a prearranged place at an agreed time. By these means I think that this officer was relieved of a little of the torture of his impending court martial. At the latter I gave my medical evidence and left, as I had already received a posting order to join No. 64 General Hospital in Alexandria. I learned later that the officer had been found not guilty.

April 6 1941, RAMC Base Depot, MEF

My dear Mum and Dad,

As you will see I've changed my address for good and all. I'm sorry to say I've said goodbye to No. 6 and am now awaiting posting to another unit. It's a way they seem to have in the army if they can muck you up they will. It all happened because of a court martial. I am called to give some quite irrelevant medical evidence, and because of that as a court martial takes precedence over everything else in the army, I am not allowed to leave the country, however urgent the requirement for surgeons may be until it is cleared up. As you probably gather from the news my old unit is likely to be shifted, I have been replaced, and am now clicking my heels doing next to damn all... .Perhaps when it's finished I shall be able to get a nice little surgical team in Yugoslavia if I start a little agitation, and as Buxton [Consultant Orthopaedic Surgeon from King's College Hospital] is out here I have one rather strong wire to pull.

I am staying in a delightful mess at the minute. In what I consider this pretty awful country here is a patch that looks just like an English garden in summer time. Of course it's getting quite hot now, and here at much expense of rather precious water is a green lawn. A rare enough sight, with masses of English flowers – antirrhinums, stock, roses and all the rest of them. It is really lovely. But again just outside this patch of green and colours is the interminable sand. However

I would not have missed coming out here for anything and soon I'm sure I shall be up to the hilt in work...

30th April 1941 No. 64 General Hospital MEF

Dear Mum and Dad

This form of letter is a new innovation. It is photographed from the original out here, reduced to the size of a postage stamp, sent to England and enlarged to the size in which you receive it. I received your last card. Did you get my second cable?

I am very happy in my new job and in view of the fact that my old unit has not yet started to function I am glad I was transferred, because I have a real lot of work to do here not just the hack work of war surgery, but other stuff as well.

How are you all at home? There are many occasions when I wish I was back, but I am afraid that will be some time yet.

Love Stanley

Nowhere could there have been a happier service hospital or one set in more delightful surroundings. On the edge of the town, overlooking the blue Mediterranean, it had taken over a school in the grounds of which wooden huts had been erected to give added accommodation, so that nearly fifteen hundred beds were available. Its gardens were purple with bougainvillaea and red with jacaranda and in the centre of its quadrangle was a lawn as green and fresh as any to be found in England. No place could have been more restful to men coming back wounded from the desert, no hospital surroundings more conducive to recovery and convalescence. Rarest of all was a sports field. In addition, a first-class concert hall was among the amenities with which this school, now a hospital, was provided.

It must not be imagined that every hospital was so happily sited.

Not many miles away, close to the delta of the Nile, railway sidings, roads, water supplies and sanitation had already been organised in a waste of sand prior to the establishment of a hospital there. Thousands of pounds had been spent when it was suddenly realised by some medical officers that the local population had a higher 'splenic index' than most places in Egypt. This index, arrived at by ascertaining what percentage of the people possessed enlarged spleens on palpating their abdomens, indicates the prevalence of malaria in a certain area. But already the initial preparations were completed. A hospital had to go there. It was rumoured that an attempt had been made to foist the site and the mosquitoes on to the Australians, and that they had taken one look and laughed at the 'pommy bastards' thinking they could get away with that one. So a British hospital was duly sent there, but fortunately the day came when an Indian hospital required a site. The British hospital was therefore moved and the white elephant, again, along with the mosquitoes, was adroitly disposed of.

In later months, another hospital was erected not far outside Tobruk. It was laid out on the side of a slope. On a fine day it was ideal, but whoever had chosen the situation had forgotten that every day in the desert is not sunny and still. This little area soon showed itself to be the meeting place of all the winds that blew from the four quarters of the earth. Whenever there was a dust storm, which was frequently, there you could see it at its very worst, playfully sweeping in and out of the tents and buildings of No. 1 Military Hospital at Tobruk and finally engulfing it in an impenetrable dust cloud. Moreover, in the late autumn and winter when heavy rains came to the desert, all the miniature torrents joyfully rushed through the new encampment, flooding wards, isolating tents in a sea of mud and water and making the roads through the hospital so impassable that trucks and ambulances sank axle-deep and had to be dug or towed out of the mire. It was not a happy choice, this site, but once started nothing was going to stop the completion of the project. Many were the medical officers and patients who bitterly cursed the 'high-up' who had chosen this of all places when not a few miles away was a hospital building that had been used with efficiency throughout the siege of Tobruk. Small wonder that the hospital was commonly known as the 'Folly'.

At Alexandria, however, the almost perfect site and buildings were available for a service hospital. Unless a building is designed as a hospital it is quite obvious it can never be perfect, but for the purposes of conversion a school is the next best thing. There are large classrooms and dormitories readily altered into wards, administrative offices and storerooms available, and baths and sanitation and heating and water supplies already laid on, making the organisation and running of the hospital so much easier.

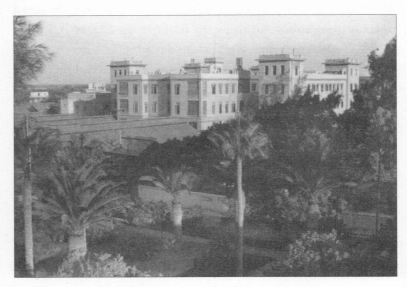

No. 64 General Hospital, Alexandria – formerly Victoria College.

It was a unique hospital in another way. It had been set up at the very beginning of the war as a combined military and naval hospital under a RAMC commanding officer with nurses and doctors from both services. Most of the junior naval officers when I arrived had already served in ships and of these a large number were survivors of vessels which had been sunk. It could have been a place where service rivalries and prejudices led to differences enough to interfere with the smooth running of the hospital. Instead, there could not have been a happier and more united staff, and it was to the then commanding officer, Colonel Melvin, that this unity was largely due. We were all very proud of the good name of No. 64 General Hospital.

Thousands upon thousands of officers and men from all over the British Empire passed through its wards, and many will still have with them, in spite of all the tragedy and suffering of war, appreciative and sometimes fond memories of days spent there. They will know that no effort was spared not only in their actual medical care but also in trying to improve their food and make their convalescent stage as comfortable and pleasant as was humanly possible. Some will remember the visits of Alice Delysia, when she sang to them in ward and concert hall. They will remember her sweetness and her charm, and the exquisite agony as memory, stirred by her songs, brought back a world of loveliness and beauty, filled with the happiness of the past and the hopes of the future; a world far away from war and horror. Others will think of a day when Josephine Baker entertained them, entrancing them so that at the end of each song it was an appreciable time before they could bring themselves to applaud and so destroy the magic spell that she had woven. There were many gifted performers, including a concert party of local residents who year in, year out travelled round entertaining the wounded and sick troops. These artistes brought amusement and diversion to thousands. They were working, as everyone else in the hospital was, surgeons, physicians, sisters and orderlies, to heal minds and bodies ravaged by war.

Surgery and medicine were essential, but a positive attitude and peace of mind were equally necessary if a patient was to recover his health rapidly and completely, and these we tried to promote.

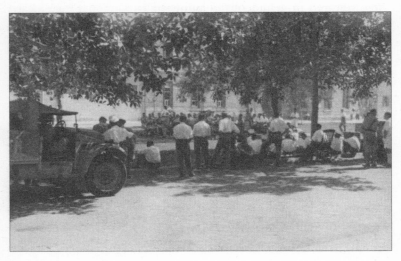

Outside the hospital.

In other respects this hospital at Alexandria was different from most in that it served a dual purpose by virtue both of its situation and because it was both naval and military in character. Not only was it a large base hospital taking cases that had mostly received preliminary treatment in the forward surgical units in the desert, but it also served as an initial treatment centre for the casualties from the fleet, with the result that seldom was it anything but busy.

In addition to the general surgical and medical work carried out by any hospital, it was the policy in the army to assign a speciality to each so that cases of a similar type could be gathered together in one or more units. This allowed a hospital to become especially expert in the nursing and treatment of certain cases, and physicians and surgeons particularly skilled in that particular branch of work were employed to deal almost solely with such injuries. Thus there were centres for the treatment of eye injuries, and hospitals especially concerned with plastic work at which soldiers who had been disfigured beyond recognition by wounds to the face were restored from hideous ghastliness to something very nearly approaching normality. Other specialities included head injuries and bone injuries, and it was for the latter that No. 64 General Hospital was one of the two centres in Egypt.

Each of the specialities required appropriate equipment and methods of treatment for their success. In the case of orthopaedic surgery, where gunshot wounds may have destroyed and disintegrated large areas of soft tissue and bony structures, the patient was faced with the prospect of months of immobilisation in bed. Special beds were necessary in order to ease nursing and provide cushioning and support so that the danger of sores developing when the patient's strength and resistance were reduced to low ebb by the prolonged sepsis of his wounds was minimal. Other apparatus was attached to each bed so that traction could readily be applied. And because of the months that lay ahead for the wounded man, during which his general morale had to be maintained and supported, his surroundings were made as pleasant and cheerful as was possible. With this in mind, a brick building was constructed with a large veranda on to which beds could readily be wheeled. This was off the other ranks' wards, and watching a cricket match, seeing the passers-by and knowing ordinary life was going on made all the difference to the monotony. The officers, on the other hand, were less fortunate because in the construction of their separate small wards no one had remembered that the orthopaedic bed is wider than the average hospital type, and all the doorways were just those few inches too narrow to allow the beds to be pushed through; so they had to remain confined in their rooms without that small change of environment that meant so much.

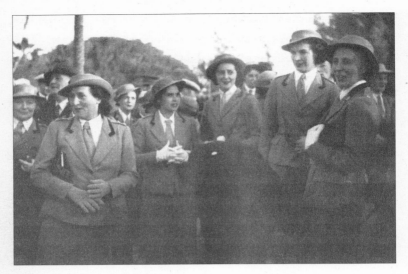

A nurses' outing in Alexandria.

The adequate treatment of fracture cases demanded a large physiotherapy department and here in Alexandria one equal to any in England was established. Regular massage and periodic electrical stimulation of muscles grown weak with disease were of the greatest importance in maintaining some semblance of normal tone and structure, so that when the patient was finally allowed out of bed, his convalescence was not marred by the muscle wastage that would otherwise have taken place.

When a limb has been immobilised for weeks on end, all the joints tend to stiffen and contract. The minimisation of this and the restoration of their movement when all the controlling splints have been removed needs a high degree of skilled physiotherapy and this, as never before in wartime, was at hand. At first the few experts from the regular ranks of the army and navy had been responsible for this work, but as the numbers of patients requiring treatment increased, their strength was augmented by teams of physiotherapists sent from England.

Patients need work to do when they are in hospital for long periods and to this end an organised workshop was set up. Those who were convalescent could go along and occupy themselves on lathes doing carpentry or woodwork, whereas to those still in bed the arts of making toys, binding books, weaving rugs or scarves, or working in leather were taught so that the time in which a patient could dwell upon his injuries and become introspective concerning his disabilities was reduced as far as possible. The deadly monotony of life, where empty day followed empty day, where the progress of a week seemed so slow to a patient who had nothing else to do but to lie and think, was minimised. There was little gloom on any of the wards in spite of the awful nature of so many of the men's wounds and when the time came for them to get up, all worries and thoughts about their injuries were lost in the thrill and excitement of once more being able to walk about, however limited their initial progress may have been.

Among the most terrible of all the injuries were those due to burns, and of the casualties from the many ships that were lost in keeping the Mediterranean open and in relieving the beleaguered garrisons at Tobruk and Malta, burns victims constituted a high proportion. Being enveloped in a sea of burning oil or a blast of superheated steam from a damaged vessel could cause these cruel injuries. From the army too these casualties came, often unfortunately in a worse state than their naval comrades. When a tank caught fire and its crew leapt out or were dragged away from the burning wreck, the natural and only thing to do was to roll on the ground in an endeavour to extinguish the flames. From that point of view it was sometimes successful, but in the process all the raw, burned areas of the man's body became coated with the sand and dirt of the desert, meaning that early infection of his wounds was inevitable. In the case of the sailor, the salt seawater was probably as good a first-aid dressing as anything.

113

The treatment of the severely burned man was formidable and problematic. Initially, during the first few hours after injury, there was little that could be done except to combat the element of shock which could so easily overwhelm him. He lay cold and clammy, perhaps almost pulseless, in that state between death and life in which appreciation and understanding of his surroundings was hazy and unreal. Only with transfusions – pint after pint run into his veins – could he be brought slowly back from that halfway stage. Then, when once again he was alive, both he and all those who looked after him were faced with the battle, uphill and often prolonged, to save his life.

From all the burned areas of his body, plasma – the almost colourless part of the blood – starts to ooze, and with it are lost the proteins, salts and fluids that he needs to support life. These can partially be replaced by transfusions, and the loss reduced by treatment, but in spite of all this, sometimes you see him slipping away, slowly, inevitably. There is an ache in your heart and you feel numb and powerless. You want to cry out, 'Why can't I do something to stop this – this victory of death over youth – this triumph over anything I can do.'

Perhaps among patients similarly hurt you try different methods. Some you may treat with aniline dyes to try and stop the ooze of plasma, some with constant nursing in a bath of saline, others with powdered sulphanilamide, searching always to turn away defeat. But no matter what is done, if the initial injury has destroyed more than a certain percentage of the covering skin surface of the body, you nearly always fight a losing battle.

Even when the first battle is won, a new danger in the form of sepsis often appears, threatening to overwhelm the patient with toxaemia; this was especially so with the army patients whose burns had been contaminated with germs from the desert dust. Penicillin is now a powerful weapon in the prevention and treatment of this complication, but before 1944 hardly any of this drug was available and other methods had to be applied. Then, finally, when this danger has been overcome and it is obvious that the wounded man will get better, a further problem comes along to trouble the surgeon. Burns scar the tissues so that left alone they tighten and contract. Fingers may be pulled down into the palm, and a claw-shaped travesty of a hand remains to replace something that was wonderful in all the intricate movements that it could perform; faces may be so disfigured with contracture that they become hideous and pathetic. But these tragedies can be averted by skin grafting, plastic surgery and patient physiotherapy, and in the specialised plastic surgical units of the RAMC patients learned that even though months of treatment lay ahead, there was no cause for despair. They would be made well, hands and fingers would once again be full of use and cleverness, faces once more express character and emotion, smile with happiness and love and sadden with the sorrows that come to trouble life.

To me it is an extraordinary thing that as soon as a war comes, the natural horror with which bloodshed and death are viewed by the average layman diminishes as he takes off his civilian clothes and dons a uniform. In fact, perhaps nature protects him more kindly than she does a medical officer. Induce a person to watch even the most minor operation in peacetime and he will probably faint or be sick. But not so in war. I well remember when I was a ship's surgeon in the Far East, before the war, asking one of the officers to help me with an operation. The third officer volunteered, but we had hardly started when he slumped to the floor; and yet I am sure that had his ship been hit in wartime he would have been one of the first to bandage and help any of his wounded crew without experiencing any queer feelings whatsoever. So it was then with our orderlies who aided our nurses in the wards, ordinary men from all walks of life, newly recruited into the RAMC or Royal

Navy, who never flinched from the sight of the terrible injuries, the care of which was partly theirs. They were fine.

I was also always surprised that, where patients were desperately wounded and dying, when death finally came it did not seem to have as bad a psychological effect on others which one might have imagined. That was indeed fortunate because, in spite of all that poets write, death is seldom beautiful. Death should be a private affair but in a military hospital in wartime it, like life, is outstandingly public.

At the hospital in Alexandria was one large ward in which the worst septic cases were nursed. They were nursed together so that any risk of the spread of infection to clean cases in other wards should not arise. Naturally, because of the grossness of some of these men's injuries, certain of them were mortally wounded. It was a heart-breaking ward. It smelt of pus and of impending death, sickly and disgusting until one's nose learnt to ignore. In spite of all our efforts it abounded in flies. Day after day you would try to encourage those whom in your heart you knew no encouragement could save. Perhaps the tears that sometimes filled your eyes belied the brave words of hope on your lips. It was not easy in such circumstances to hide one's feelings.

Sometimes screens would be put around the bed as a man started his last journey. But all the time the ward would be loud with talk and the wireless would blaze away, and only when the bar was crossed and a guard came to carry the Union Jack-draped body away, were the radio and the talk silenced. But only for a few brief moments. The talk would start again, a little quietly at first, and then the wireless would be switched on once more. In a few minutes the ward would be back to its normal self, except for one empty bed. It was better that way than that dark despondency, futile and damaging, be allowed to descend.

Sometimes, however, even in this ward, life would steal slowly back into bodies so torn and injured that they seemed barely to have any basis for existence. There was a South African sergeant, whose name was Norse. He had been cruelly wounded by an anti-personnel shell filled with pieces of scrap metal, some of which had penetrated his abdomen and his chest. For months he hovered. He had thirteen operations in all and perhaps at times he saw despair in the faces of his doctors and his nurses. 'Don't give up, doc,' he once said. 'If you do your best I'll do mine and I'll be all right.' Determination to live makes all the difference between success and failure and one day the sergeant was well enough to be sent down to South Africa. Now he is back farming, doing all that he did before the war.

There was another patient, a New Zealander named Turner. He developed gas gangrene, which happily was rare among the wounded in the Middle East. He lost an arm, but in spite of this the disease spread up to his shoulder, on to his chest wall and down to his flank. Toxaemia was steadily overwhelming him and, in an effort to do something rather than the other alternative of watching him slowly die, we slashed open all the infected tissues with wide incisions and excised what we could. To our intense relief he started to recover from that day. The sickly, sweet smell of the gangrene cleared away from his bed. Instead of being drowsy with the toxins from the infection, he became alive and well.

There was no sense of pride in cases like these. There was just the feeling of great relief and gratefulness that life had turned back at the very point of departure. Somewhere far away you knew that there would be happy hearts and tears of thankfulness. They were not just men; they were the beloved of many. They were sons and husbands, sweethearts and lovers. They were life and hope itself to those who cherished them across the seas.

About that time I wrote to my parents:

24 May 1941
Major S. O. Aylett
No. 64 General Hospital, MEF

My dear Mum and Dad – I received your 10th letter but I think about 5 have gone astray.

I am now working very hard. Events in the desert and in Crete have brought this about. It is really a heartrending and tragic sight. I have two particularly dreadful wards. The one is a septic ward. You go into this enormous ward of 100 beds and the first thing that strikes you is the stink of pus, of faeces and of urine and that of the foul discharge of stinking wounds. Then you become conscious of the flies. Flies everywhere, black with flies all feeding on the discharge of the wounds and all the other filth they find. You can 'flit', you can swat a dozen each whack with your swatter, and it makes no difference. Then you become aware of the blasting of the radio and perhaps at the other end of the ward the stertorous breathing of patients about to pass into the great beyond. Suddenly the breathing stops. Screens are drawn round, the talking ceases and someone turns off the radio. Then the mortuary party appears with a Union Jack and with this draped over the body another chapter is ended. The talking starts again, at first rather self-consciously as if each wonders whose turn it will be next, and then the hum of talk becomes louder and the wireless is turned on again and the ward returns to its abnormal normal.

Pus and filth, rotting bodies. Oh, how tragic. If you have a chance, go and see *Gone with the Wind* and in that film you will see my septic ward in this year of the Lord's grace and goodness nineteen hundred and forty-one.

Then I go along to my burns ward where I have been most

of the day. We get a lot of burns, the result of ships on fire and petrol and oil explosions. There you will see men with skin burned off most of their bodies, swathed in bandages, looking like so many mummies. Now and then you will hear the shriek of uncontrollable agony and you will see some delirious patients fighting to get out of bed.

Don't think that I am depressed. Far from it. I just thought that you would like a picture of what our hospital is really like.

My love to you always and take care of yourselves.

With love,

Stanley

Such was the life in our hospital in its frequent busy periods, when sleep came when it could no longer be resisted and meals when the opportunity arose. But big battles did not go on in the desert for weeks on end. Both sides wore themselves out and had to regroup and replenish their numbers, replace their wrecked tanks, guns and lorries. Piles of ammunition, mines, petrol and other stores had to be assembled in preparation for the next onslaught and in these periods work in our hospital correspondingly slackened. We too occupied this time in preparing for the next wave of carnage.

Wounded prisoners of war were nursed in separate wards with minimum security yet none attempted to escape, although Alexandria contained hundreds whose sympathies were with the Axis. These wards were newly built wooden huts but with the influx of Italian and Libyan wounded that followed Wavell's destruction of their armies, they had become infested with bed bugs. Whatever we did we were never able to eradicate these revolting pests. We could burn the skirting boards until they smouldered, spray with all our available insecticides, put each bed-foot into a tin containing paraffin to stop these evil 'mahogany flats', as they were called, crawling up from the floor, but then they seemed to drop from the roof. We kept them under control but they were always there, especially at night. Then our nurses rarely escaped the weals the bites of these insects raised on their legs. Only an immediate bath and the laundering of all their clothes prevented the introduction of these bugs into their own quarters.

Feeling between Italians and Germans ran high. They were more like enemies than allies. On one occasion a severely wounded Italian required several pints of blood. I did not see why, on this occasion, when in the ward were several very lightly wounded Germans, they should not donate their blood. When it was explained, however, that this was for one of their Italian friends, they refused.

I sent for the interpreter. Through him I pointed out that we had given our own blood to help save many of their comrades. If they, in their turn, refused to give blood for their allies we would certainly refuse point blank to give any more to our enemies. It was only then that they decided to give blood for this desperately ill Italian.

In May, King Peter of Yugoslavia visited the hospital. After the invasion of his country by the Germans and the destruction of Belgrade, the Nazi armies had entered the ruined capital mid-April. Immediately all those who had played any part in deposing the pro-German regent Paul had been sought and those who were caught either shot or hanged. The king escaped through Greece to Egypt but his chief of air staff, one of those mainly responsible for the coup, had stayed in the city for a few days evading those searching for him. Disguised, he had managed to take photographs of some of the German atrocities. Finally, he and some other officers had managed to seize a plane and escape. This was hit by anti-aircraft fire and General Simovic was shot through the leg. The plane reached Alexandria where it crash-landed and the occupants came under my care. It was these whom King Peter had come to visit.

The film that had been brought out of Yugoslavia was developed, and I was given copies of the prints with a request that I show them to as many people as possible so they would realise what occupation by the Nazis really meant. This I did. They were pictures of atrocity, which shocked all who saw them.

9

NON-MEDICAL DUTIES IN A GENERAL HOSPITAL

JUNE 1941–FEBRUARY 1942

Recreational activities; breaks in Alexandria;
visit to the Holy Land

O ur duties as medical officers, whether in the Royal Navy or the RAMC, were not only to care for the wounded and sick. The hospital was a very large one with a complement of several hundred men responsible for its many services. It was going to be there for a long time, certainly for as long as the war in the Middle East continued and for such time as the Mediterranean had to be kept safe for British shipping. The end could not be foreseen and this large community needed the provision of efficient social services and recreational facilities. Most of the other ranks, NCOs and petty officers, too, would serve their whole time in the same hospital.

Sports – cricket, tennis, football and hockey – were organised and a dance band formed from the many talents of our men. There was a library and a gramophone club to run, a magazine to be edited, and a host of other activities to supervise. An officer had to be in charge of the company messing and to ensure that the extra funds available from the unit accounts were spent to the best possible advantage in the provision of food additional to army rations. There were bars to supervise, accounts to be prepared and, at the end of each quarter, audited. We were not at a loss to know what to do when our hospital went through one of its slack periods.

Each of these essential sidelines to the medical work of a large hospital was run by a committee elected by the other ranks. An officer appointed by the CO had the ultimate responsibility for co-ordinating wishes and ideas and for making a success of each particular enterprise. Guided by these committees the social life of the hospital prospered. Not only did they assemble a much-sought-after dance band and a very good football side, but under the direction of a most talented officer, Captain Ian Mclver, they also produced a Christmas show which gave several public performances in the town.

All these activities might seem very remote from the vitally important purpose of a medical unit, but in point of fact they were all a part of it. The work of a nursing orderly was hard and often monotonous, as it was carried out in one particular ward. For hour after hour he was in contact with the same often desperately ill patients. Only if he came back from his off-duty hours fresh in mind could he do justice to those for whom he was helping to care. All the sports and hobbies available played a part in maintaining enthusiasm, which, at times of prolonged contact with the ugliness of gross wounds and of death itself, might otherwise have wavered. It must be remembered that the large majority of these fine men had had little or no contact with sickness before joining their service; they had had none of the years of training of the nurse or doctor. They were swept into the life of a hospital by the demands of war with the minimum of preparation.

In addition, the social side of the hospital brought officers and men into closer understanding with each other, and the team spirit essential for success in our professional work was assured. Our own mess consisted of both army and naval officers. Rank meant very little to us, as we were all doctors. Chance had made of one a colonel and of another a captain. The fortunes of war may have designated the general practitioner senior to the consultant whom in peacetime he used to ask to see his patients. On the other hand, an experienced doctor of many years' standing and wearing distinguished medals from the last war might find himself ranked below a very recently qualified medical officer who was fortunate enough to have achieved a higher professional degree. It was all rather topsy-turvy but it was only the very few who bore any grudge. It was the ability of the officer rather than the number of pips upon his shoulders or gold rings around his cuffs that we came to respect. Our salute as we passed our seniors was really not to the officer but to the king whose uniform he wore: most times we could acknowledge both with respect.

We lived together as month followed month, bound by our work and by the force of the personalities of some of our members who wove our individualism into unity. To achieve for our patients the best possible level of comfort and contentment was the aim of our concerted effort.

To this end, the work of the president of a mess and the mess committee was of considerable importance. It might seem a waste of professional time, but even in a doctors' mess someone had to supervise the cooking and the food, especially in a country such as Egypt where native servants were employed in order to economise on manpower. Someone still had to see that the laundry came and went, without too many losses, or too many tears and holes, that rooms and bathrooms were cleaned, and that accounts were kept in order and overhead costs were reduced to a minimum. These were a few of the chores of any household and the comfort of a mess depended largely on how well they were carried out. If they were supervised badly, a mess would become slovenly, and if the officers' mess of any unit is poorly run, the unit as a whole is not first class. In Alexandria we were fortunate in having officers to whom these mundane duties were not laborious and wearisome and we benefited accordingly.

The bar was naturally the focal point of the mess and behind it for many months serving out the drinks was Toni. He was a medical orderly in the Italian navy and had been picked up when his ship was sunk. He bubbled over with high spirits and exuberance in his new job, which was so similar to his work in the bar he owned in Naples. We all had invitations to go and visit it after the war and an uproarious time he would have given us. Only when he remembered his *bambinos* did tears come into his eyes, but thoughts of his wife did not seem to affect him as much. One day, just before Christmas, as he was a non-combatant, orders came for his repatriation. Tears streamed from his eyes and he embraced us all before leaving, insisting that we should come and see him. Sadly I lost his address in that wonderful city.

When I first arrived at the hospital, a Greek was employed part-time to look after the accounts of the mess and to supervise the catering and the wines and spirits' side of the bar. I soon began to have grave suspicions as to the honesty and integrity of this particular civilian and wondered how much was disappearing from the mess funds. The president was an officer senior to myself and when I approached him he told me he thought things were all right. For health reasons this officer was subsequently sent home and I was elected as his successor.

It was a large mess, often numbering over seventy officers, and as I went through the accounts with him before he left I noticed considerable irregularities. I am quite good at figures and reached the conclusion that the funds had been relieved of over seven hundred and fifty pounds, which in those days was a large amount of money. The Greek gentleman concerned was sent for and I asked him to explain the many discrepancies. He denied them all, left the room and we never saw him again. I was concerned as to what to do. It was quite apparent that I should have reported these discrepancies, but this would have involved a big enquiry and the officer concerned, who was completely blameless of the irregularities except in his lack of any financial sense, would have been held responsible and perhaps his return to the UK cancelled. I called a meeting of the whole of the mess and told them of the position. I told them that by increasing the mess charges by a few piastres each day, by lowering the standard of the food a little and increasing the bar charges this deficit could be converted into a small profit. My suggestion was accepted. I then ran the messing and the bar and when I left the unit we were back in the black. A surgeon's lot in the army was not only about surgery.

To our colonel, Colonel Melvin, much of the success of this unit was due. No suggestion for improvement was too small for his consideration and reasoned judgement, and no red tape that could be broken was allowed to hinder the wellbeing and comfort of the patient or any member of his staff. It was his contention that if for months and perhaps years on end his staff, doctors, nurses and orderlies were to keep fit in a climate that at times was humid and oppressive, and in work that was arduous and filled with sadness, they must have periodic leaves. There was to be no question as to whether the man wanted his leave or not, he was to take it. He could of course stay in the hospital and spend his days bathing, playing tennis or otherwise occupying himself, but for a few days he was not allowed to go into the wards.

He was very wise this colonel. In looking after the very ill something more than just technical skill is given to the patient by the doctor. There is discretion, the weighing up of every aspect of his illness, the assessing of what is in his best interests. There is no room for error and the worry does not end when the doctor leaves the patient, but rather it goes with him and remains until finally it can be dispelled. Then, in addition, there is something indefinable, something above all this that the doctor tries to give to the desperately ill. Perhaps it is hope, perhaps it is courage, perhaps it is a part of his very soul that is passed on in a last endeavour to make the patient well. There is something, however, that he gives, beyond scientific explanation, beyond assessment, beyond physical and mental ability, and when, as in war, he is constantly in contact with the very ill, he becomes tired beyond the measure that can be assessed. Only by going away periodically from the hospital atmosphere can he continue to do his best. So it was, too, with all who were concerned with the nursing and care of these desperate cases.

July 9th 1941 No. 64 Gen Hospital MEF

My dear Mum and Dad,
Your letters are by now arriving. The mails really are extraordinarily good considering all circumstances and one letter I had from you was salvaged from the sea.

Things are generally satisfactory. Buxton pays periodic visits to the hospital in his capacity as consulting orthopaedic surgeon so I see him about once a month. I am anxious to get to a unit which is a little farther removed from the base, and I am sure that when a good suitable CCS turns up I shall be leaving here...

As you've probably heard on the wireless we have been getting pretty severe air raids. The trouble of course is that most of the native houses in this city would almost fall down if there was a severe shower of rain so that you can imagine what bombs do and so proportionately the casualties are very heavy...

I think today I had the highest compliment paid to me that I have ever received. There is always a certain amount of friction between the Aussies and the British, and in many ways the former haven't much time for us. Of course this is all due to misunderstandings, and individually they are very charming. I had operated on two of them and they were helping having convalesced in the theatre. After I thanked them and they said, we don't mind doing anything for you, Sir. Coming from Australians I felt well at least I've helped to promote some better understanding between ourselves.

The sun shines all and every day. How nice it would be to have a real good downpour, or even a real good London fog. Still I'll have to wait for that.

Goodbye for the present.

Love from Stanley.

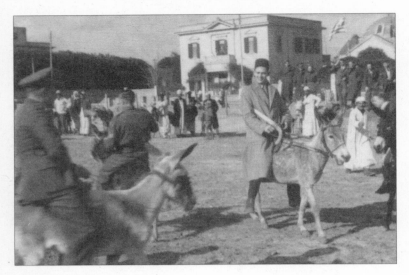

A burdened donkey.

★   ★   ★

Alexandria, in spite of the constant war that was being waged a few hours' motor drive away, was a glamorous and beautiful place. In the shimmering sun and in the freshness of the early morning, it was a poor soul who could not find beauty and rest in the enormous sweep of the bay beyond which the Mediterranean sparkled in a million dancing lights that flashed from its dark-blue surface. There was rest from war and escape from sickness, lying on its sands and bathing in the gentle warmth of that sea. Then, when the sun had passed its height and the great heat of the day abated, there were sports to play, of every type, in conditions of near perfection.

For those who wanted to wander idly, there were shops in abundance to visit and admire, filled with all the luxuries that were disappearing from our world at home. There were the treasures of the East too – carpets from Persia, heavy and exquisite damasks and silks from Syria, and gold and silver work from the craftsmen of

Egypt – and, for those who wished to escape back into antiquity, there were the relics of a day when Cleopatra ruled and held court for Antony.

Then as the light crept out of the sky and the red and gold horizon gradually lost its flame, becoming pastel with quiet colour, the coolness of the evening descended, refreshing and perfect. Below the deep purple of the heavens, set with diamond stars, stretched the tranquil sea, now dark and indistinct save where a thousand moonbeams were reflected from its surface. Perhaps in the evening light you could look at a face beside you and see another heaven there, one that in its serenity and beauty dispelled all the bitter hurt and disillusionment of war. For a few hours the world had left you, it was remote and far away. Soon you would have to return, but with a radiant memory of happiness that neither time nor the burdens of life could ever take away.

Sometimes, in the evenings, we would go down to the Excelsior in the centre of the city. This dance hall would always be packed. Officers on leave from the desert or from their ships or planes – Australians, New Zealanders, Rhodesians and South Africans, British and Greeks and others too were there. And there were girls from all the branches of the women's services. We drank sparingly and danced excessively. The trumpeter played and the floor shook as the piercing, searing notes of 'In The Mood' urged us on. Then we would watch the cabaret of belly dancers, take the floor ourselves once more, and dance until the closing number. Perhaps for many this was their ball before Waterloo.

Palestine and Luxor were two other places where troops could spend their leave periods and in so far as was possible the army made every arrangement to allow visits to these areas. When I took one trip I had been ill with jaundice, an illness which was almost epidemic at the time, affecting hundreds upon hundreds of men serving in the Middle East. After a stay in my own hospital, during which I was sadly over-spoiled, I was given a few days' convalescent leave and decided to visit the Holy Land. The Palestine Express, which was due to start from the Canal at midnight and eventually trundled off about three hours late, may have been misnamed, but when it was filled with leave parties it was a happy train, however many hours it took to roll its way towards Palestine. Long journeys meant nothing when one had been in the army a while. As a civilian it was reasonable to think twice before travelling hundreds of miles for a few fleeting hours of holiday, but one became so used to covering great distances in the most unpleasant of circumstances that nothing was thought of it.

The train had started so late that soon the outlines of the dunes emerged from the darkness as the sun rose. The train followed an historic route along which the armies of Allenby had passed. At first it crossed wastes of featureless sand where black-outlined camels and their huddled drivers plodded slowly, making the most of the relative cool of the early morning. Gradually the yellowed drabness changed to welcome green, scrub gave place to palm trees and orange groves, and in the distance hills, hazy and blue, were visible. The small villages and towns through which we passed seemed cleaner and more ordered than those in Egypt and the primitive means of cultivation were largely left behind. Wearily the train drew towards Lydda, the junction town for Jerusalem, for which city most were bound, and then pressed onward again towards Haifa and from thence into Syria.

I got out at Haifa because I wanted first to visit the fortress town of Acre, centre of so many sieges in the past. Outside its fortifications, the armies of Napoleon were halted in their endeavour to conquer the Middle East as a step towards realising his dream of a French-Indian Empire. There they waited, for reinforcements arriving by sea, but that help never arrived. Their transports were sunk by a small British squadron that lay just off the coast and the dream ended in retreat before a force of Turkish soldiers and British sailors. Yet in a way how mighty a triumph had been this march of the French army out of Egypt up towards Syria. A desert of sand had been crossed and all the problems of water supply, transportation and disease which a modern army were finding so enormous had seemingly been overcome by the military prowess of nearly a hundred and fifty years ago. Perhaps the route was strewn with the bodies of those who had indeed been stricken with illness or with thirst, so that the thinness of their numbers helped to halt them, but it was those few British ships that had really robbed this venture of success. Part of the old town and the castle, then used as a prison, still remained. Further back in the centuries, in the time of the Crusaders, Richard Coeur de Lion had laid siege to this strategic prize, finally capturing it from the forces of Saladin. The remains of a Crusaders' chapel still served as a monument to another dream of the past.

The bus wound up the curved road from Haifa to Jerusalem, to the lovely old walled city, through whose gates the apostles had passed and Jesus had ridden on the journey that would lead him to the cross. The roads inside the city were narrow, sloping down and shaded from the sun by ancient and torn canvas stretched between the houses, which leaned ever closer to each other with the passing centuries. Again, all the craftsmen of the Middle East were hammering their silver and their gold, weaving their carpets and sewing their exquisite materials, and drinking small cups of hot dark sweet coffee, while burdened donkeys staggered under their loads along the steep and ill-paved streets. I made my way to the Wailing Wall and watched as every Jew who passed stopped to touch and kiss in reverence these stones imbued with thousands of years of his history and to intone a traditional prayer. Close by was the Mosque of Omah where a different prophet was worshipped and where, after washing, his followers knelt and turned towards

Mecca in not dissimilar prayer. An eternal presence was very real in this city, but men had fought and killed in their millions over the identity of that eternal presence.

We went to the sepulchre and paid our shillings to get in and they felt like the thirty pieces of silver. 'Them that sold and them that bought' still used the temples like market places. We were told all the arguments for believing that this cave was holy ground from which Christ had risen and we left in silent thought and veneration. We did not know that a few hundred yards further on was a similar cave claiming that only it was genuine.

In Bethlehem, five miles south of Jerusalem, a guide, who you have not asked for or indeed employed, takes you to the Church of the Nativity. You bend your head under the low lintel and descend a stone stairway to the actual place of the divine birth. The walls of the stairway are lined with wooden boards painted to look like tapestry. The guide tells us that in the past real tapestries were hung there but clashing religious sects set fire to them so often that they have been replaced. It is very dark near the birthplace but the guide soon overcomes this by seizing a large candle from the altar to illuminate a hollow depression in the stone floor. You feel you want to run away and keep your vision of this holy setting intact, remembering Christ's birthplace as a manger, fresh and simple with the smell of hay.

We went back to Jerusalem, walked up the Via Dolorosa and paid out our coins at the various Stations of the Cross. Great faith and belief could perhaps ignore all that was temporal in this city and discover solace in these places of Christ's teaching, but it was hard to do.

Outside the old walled city, the modern Jerusalem offered all the attractions which go into making a good leave, for when the soldier had tired of wandering down ancient alleys and streets where the houses almost touched and the sunshine rarely penetrated, he could return to good hostels and hotels, to cinemas and dance clubs. Many went down to the Dead Sea to bathe in this large salt lake over a thousand feet below the level of the Mediterranean, where it is difficult to prevent one's legs from shooting above the surface so great is the density of the water. It is arid, hot and barren there and, except for the novelty of trying to swim in an inland sea that resents your presence and perpetually tries to throw you out, it was a precious working day largely wasted.

10

INCIDENTS AT THE HOSPITAL

JUNE 1941–FEBRUARY 1942

Congeniality of the workplace; eccentric colleagues, in particular
Major Geoffrey Morley; visit to the Upper Nile

Returning to our unit at Alexandria from any leave held few
regrets. For most of us it had become far more than a hospital:
it had become our home and our life for the months or years that
circumstances dictated. It was not just a characterless institution but
also a place where great friendship underlay our routine of work
and play. For most units in the RAMC and probably in other corps,
this atmosphere existed, and I can remember only one to which it
was not a pleasure to return.

On being again among one's colleagues in a hospital back
in England, in the past, one would have been asked, 'Did you
have a nice holiday?' though you would have known they were
not deeply concerned to hear what had happened to you; but
abroad it was different. Those with whom you worked really

were interested. You showed the presents and other purchases that you had made, told where you had been, and where, when their turn came round, it was best to go and stay. There was a shop that perhaps you had found in some bazaar where silks or carpets could be purchased that were better than elsewhere. You described how for hours you had bargained and showed what finally you had bought, or you recounted the amusing incidents that had happened on your trip.

The returning officer on his side had to catch up with events in the hospital while he had been away. He had to find out what had happened to those patients whom he had left somewhat anxiously and whether there had been changes of staff during his leave. There were simple domestic matters too. Even the vagaries of our pets concerned us all. We had a cat who was extremely fond of coiling herself up into service caps left on the table outside our mess. As the caps were a mixture of blue and khaki, we were always exercised as to which she should favour when it came to giving birth to her kittens. Each of us hoped that the honour would fall to the opposite service, but the cat was a diplomatic cat, anxious to cause no disruption to our unity by petty jealousy, and when the happy event arrived she abandoned her accustomed beds and found a neutral corner in which to rear her family.

There were always the eccentricities of certain of our officers to be updated on. We had a very good surgeon, a man of young middle age who was a teetotaller. He was devoted to his wife and children and yet one night he inexplicably decided to walk round a sloping parapet that surrounded our mess, which was no more than a foot broad with a thirty-foot drop down to the road below. It was a near suicidal walk but he accomplished the feat successfully. On one particularly close evening, he was coming home when he decided he was far too hot. It was a matter of moments before he was continuing his walk naked save for his shoes and socks. That such a natural means of cooling off should cause any comment from his more convention-bound colleagues amazed him.

We had another officer, Major Geoffrey Morley, of whom we were very fond and whose activities were always a source of wonder. He had had an amazing career. During the last war he had become a midshipman in the Royal Navy, but had soon been invalided out owing to constant seasickness. He was still underage for enlistment so, somehow or other, he made his way to Italy where he joined the Italian Air Force, transferring to the Royal Flying Corps as soon as he reached the necessary age. He had flown in the Near East, so he knew the country well. After the war he had become a test pilot, but following a crash, decided that he would like to live a longer life than was likely in that occupation. He determined to take up medicine and went to Australia where, in addition to qualifying, he became an authority on the native flora.

Fancy took him to Vienna, but having found that making a reasonable livelihood there was difficult for a foreigner, he stayed only until he could raise enough money to shift his home and family. Such difficulties were unlikely to present more than a very temporary embarrassment to a man of his capabilities. With finances augmented by journalism, and by money given to him by Americans for help in presenting their original theses for the University of Vienna's degrees and diplomas, he returned to England.

There was never anything ordinary about the holidays he took in the peacetime years. He had little interest in visiting places on the usual tourist trail, and on one occasion planned to drive into Eastern Europe and up into what were to become Iran and Iraq. The financial side of such a trip to the average doctor meant that it was unlikely to rise above the level of a dream, but Geoff had overcome these troubles before. He advertised seats in his car, and to his surprise had many applicants anxious to make the journey. He visited various firms who, from the advertisement point of view, were interested in his trek along rough roads and desert tracks. Special tyres that would not sink into the sand were given to him and special headlights and other fittings. All he had to do on his return was to write an article in a motor journal saying, 'Thanks to the Dunstone tyres with which the car was fitted, we did not notice the numerous potholes that would otherwise have made the journey across the desert impossible' or, 'The magnificent headlights fitted by Messrs Floodlight made night driving as easy as a daytime journey' and the firms supplying these otherwise expensive items were satisfied. So the trip was reduced to a financial level that was probably not more than the cost of a holiday down in Devon or Cornwall, and he had the thrill of travelling thousands of miles to the countries that he wished to visit.

He was a man a lot older than most of us, and he certainly did not have the appearance of one who had such a gift for getting the things in life on which he had set his heart. He looked like a three-quarter edition of Mr Pickwick, bespectacled and kindly, slightly portly, offering cheer to all those patients, officers and men with whom he worked. He spoke many languages fluently and in addition was a photographer only just below professional standard.

He had been in the RAMC in Abyssinia for some time, a country in which he was very interested. The difficulty there was getting about, but somehow a car always seemed available. Indeed, after many months the local brigadier had occasion to remind him of the uses to which army transport had to be confined. But following their lunch together after the interview, they parted the best of friends. Now other methods would have to be devised to overcome the transport difficulties. There was always a way.

At Alexandria, from no instruments, no music and no musicians, under Geoff's Aladdin-like guidance a full dance band appeared in a very short while. There was a little difficulty over a trumpeter, but from among his patients a second Louis Armstrong was discovered. The man was due to be discharged, but that would have been a disaster. On re-examination he was found, fortunately, to be suffering from a chronic complaint which was likely to take months and months to heal, if it ever did. The dance band was delighted, as were the various units to which it played, and, of course, the patient who had expected to be in hospital for a mere few days was thrilled to learn of this small ailment, the treatment for which necessitated his staying there indefinitely as a trumpeter. The colonel, during his weekly inspection, might possibly come to recognise his face and wonder why he was still there, but no doubt a rehearsal could be arranged on those mornings in order to spare the commanding officer another worry to add to those with which he was, quite possibly, already overburdened. He was with us a long time, that trumpeter, and when he finally had to appear before a medical board, well, it took place only a few days after his trouble had finally cleared up. The dance band was never quite the same when Louis Armstrong mark II departed.

In addition to his many other achievements, Geoff was an authority on lemurs and from the Cairo zoo he acquired one of these attractive animals. Apparently he had possessed one during the last war, which had shared his cockpit through most of his flying hours. He used to say that it kept him warm as he wore it, so to speak, wrapped round his neck. On one occasion the animal was the cause of an unfortunate scene as a high-handed senior officer claimed that it was an act of insubordination to salute with a chattering beast draped round one's neck, and anyhow it was not official neckwear. The incident closed with Geoff for some days being confined to barracks.

We were very fond of Mish-Mish, as the lemur was called, except when she had been drinking the dregs of the wine glasses, when she became ill-tempered and lacking in judgement. Having made a leap across the room and failing to reach her objective, entirely due to her own befuddled state, she would vent her anger on whoever was nearest, cursing and swearing and blaming it all on the unfortunate officer. However, when Mish-Mish did make a justifiable mistake and had a severe accident we were all very upset. One day we were out in a three-ton lorry that was bowling along at about forty miles an hour. Mish-Mish was with us, obviously very bored with the trip. Presumably to relieve the boredom, she decided upon some trapeze work on the crossbars that supported the canopy of the lorry. After a little loosening up, she was prepared for the big event and a great deal of chattering and squeaking announced the coming great leap through space and demanded everyone's attention. This big act was to consist of a leap from the foremost crossbar to the very rear one. Unhappily, Mish-Mish had forgotten that the lorry was travelling along quite quickly. At the end of her flight, instead of grasping the far rail, which had moved an appreciable distance forwards, she flew through the back of the lorry into thin air, cursing and swearing at the shabby trick that had been played upon her. She never forgave us, and although the day came when her bandages were taken off and she returned to the social life of the mess, there was never that atmosphere of mutual trust without which cordial relations do not flourish.

From time to time older specialists in the Middle East were relieved and returned home to the UK and the sad day came when we gave Geoff his farewell dinner. We knew we were losing a great personality. There were two routes home, one by ship around the Cape and the other by air across Africa to Lagos and thence to England by the much shortened sea trip. The latter, however, was reserved for the Very Important Persons of this life, and foolishly the RAMC had not included Geoff in the list. He had been to see the transport officer who had told him that there was not the slightest hope of him getting a passage by air either for himself or for Mish-Mish, who was accompanying him. We, however, who knew Geoff better than the army authorities, laughed at their refusal and were quite certain that when the plane took off from Cairo, both passengers would be aboard. The regular route may well have satisfied the average person, especially if he was homeward bound, but it did not come up to Geoff's standards. In the past we had seen a Lysander put at his disposal when he was going up to Cairo from Alexandria, and a man who could mobilise an aeroplane for himself – how we never knew – was most unlikely not to find a seat on a large Sunderland flying boat.

Of course, in a short while we heard from him that he was now in Lagos. By contacting the pilot of the flying boat he had somehow, by virtue of being in the Flying Corps in the last war, managed to secure a seat. When he arrived at the West African port, however, his troubles were not over. The transit camp was filled to overflowing with many high-ups anxiously and impatiently awaiting the few ships available for the second leg of the journey. A mere major in the RAMC, had he not been Geoff, might have waited there for weeks.

Within a few days of his arrival, a transport arrived to carry RAF personnel only. Seeing no reason why he should not try and avail himself of any benefit that the wings he wore might bring, he joined in the queue for embarkation and got on board, but before long his illegal presence was noted by the transport officer and he was ordered off. Foreseeing the probability of such an eventuality, he had taken particular care to have his luggage stowed in some quite inaccessible place in the hold. He naturally had to agree with the transport officer about going back ashore but insisted that his gear should go ashore with him. A long hunt ensued, but his cases could not be located, and in view of the fact that the ship was due to sail at any minute, he was finally given permission to remain on board. Major Morley went back to England the way all of us knew he would: we never heard whether Mish-Mish went with him. Some people are born to triumph over any difficulty. He, lovable and charming, was one of these.

Meanwhile, 1941 drew to a close. It had started with victories in the desert but there was some doubt as to how it would end. Each side advanced and retreated, losing strength in an advance, when communications and supply difficulties increased, and gaining in retreat as they fell back on set bases. It looked as if this pendulum war in the desert might go on indefinitely.

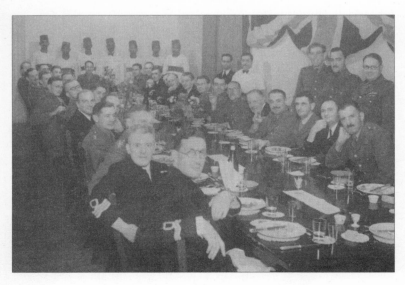

Christmas dinner at No. 64 General Hospital, 1941. (Major Morley, owner of Mish-Mish, stands on the right.)

Rommel had become something of a legend. Touring about in the desert, he had even visited a Dominion casualty clearing station (CCS), taking away those of his wounded that could be moved and thanking the doctors for looking after them.

Tobruk still resisted desperately. The supplies for its defence, as well as that of Malta, came through the Mediterranean only at the expense of high losses to the Royal Navy and the merchant service. Special high-speed ships had been sent out from England but their chances of survival were small. The battle fleet had been weakened by the loss of the *Barham*, which, struck by torpedoes, blew up and disappeared in a few minutes with the loss of over eight hundred of its crew.

One day in December, a terrific explosion shook Alexandria. Midget Italian submarines had penetrated the harbour and fixed limpet explosives on to the hulls of two battleships, the *Queen Elizabeth* and the *Valiant*, and on to that of the *Warspite*, a merchant ship. With the *Warspite* damaged, the *Elizabeth* resting on the bottom of Alexandria harbour and the *Valiant* towed into dry dock, it seemed that there was little that could prevent a powerful bombardment of the coast and a possible invasion attempt by the relatively strong Italian fleet.

The coastal batteries along the Corniche were increased as air raids on Alexandria became frequent. Most of the bombs fell on the closely packed poorer quarters of the town around the dock areas, and the mud-brick houses collapsed like toys knocked over by a child. Casualties were heavy and fear spread through the district. All day and every day thousands left to reach the open desert. Trains leaving Alexandria station were packed beyond capacity; they could not have held an extra passenger. Hanging on to the carriage doors, crowding the roofs and clinging to the buffers, they sought escape. Frightened mothers carrying their pathetic bundles of newborn infants and a straggling stream of children jostled their way through the mob outside the station. It was again the exodus caused by war, the same wild fear that had run through France and Belgium eighteen months earlier.

At the hospital we were busy with the casualties from the desert and from the sea. Our wounded German prisoners of war were often arrogant with the conviction that victory and release were not far away. It was difficult to be sympathetic towards them. True there were some exceptions but at this time the majority were treated as a duty. It was they by their insolence who destroyed any chance of building a relationship of understanding. In any hospital ward in wartime, there had to be a certain discipline, moderate and reasonable though firm. But it was the lightly wounded Nazi who tried to undermine this and by so doing put at risk the care that was ever ready and waiting to be given to his very ill comrades. Feeling between Italians and Germans ran high. The latter despised their allies as inferiors and the Italians resented this attitude, which the Germans were never at pains to hide.

Once again the bed bugs thrived in these crowded prisoner-of-war wards and the nurses suffered with the men. Again we sprayed the ward walls, used blowlamps on the crevices between the wooden planks until they scorched, and stripped the beds frequently, but we did not eliminate them, only just managing to keep them under control.

★　★　★

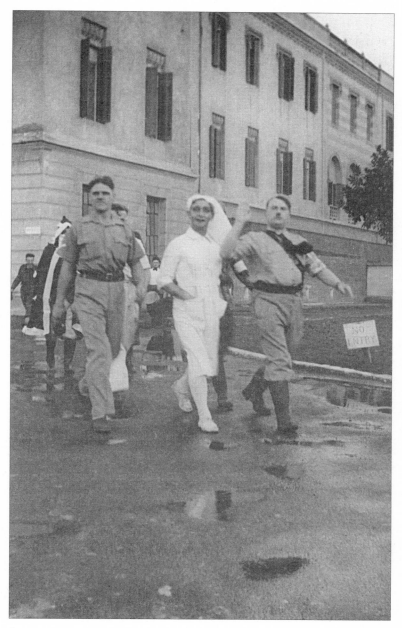

Adolf accompanying Father Christmas on his rounds, 1941.

In spite of the news, so depressing and only relieved by the knowledge that we were no longer alone but had gained two gigantic Allies in the year that was passing, Christmas came, as it does to all hospitals, cheerful and bright in spite of suffering. The sound of carols drifted through the wards, treble voices clear and fresh as the tumbling waters of a mountain stream. Christmas trees, flickering with candlelight, brought homes thousands of miles away very close.

Across the dimly lit ward, looking over the beds of his comrades, it wasn't difficult for the wounded man to see the shining and happy faces of his children. There they were, gathered round the Christmas tree, watching the candles drip their wax and pointing excitedly to the presents and the coloured glass globes decorating its branches. Yes, he could even see hanging there the presents that he had sent off months before. It wasn't hard to see his wife too, but perhaps he could not see her face quite as well as he expected. He knew it was her and that she was talking to Michael, Guy and Mary in the voice he recognised so well, telling them that perhaps next Christmas daddy would be home again. He wanted to stretch out so that he could hold her hand; he knew then that she would look round at him, smile with a tenderness and love that would make his heart ache – ache so terribly – while once again his memory of the face he knew so well grew clear. But, as he stretched out, the candles guttered and died. Those who were life itself to him had gone back across the miles, and now once more there were red blankets and white sheets, splints and bandages to limit and confine his world.

Jan. 1 1942 No. 64 General Hospital, MEF

I saw Buxton today. You will remember that when I joined the army I was not very popular at Kings. But today something must have bitten him because he was saying how scandalous and disgraceful it was that no other registrar had joined the services from Kings. So perhaps with time opinions change.

I am afraid however that any pretensions I once upon a time had of being a great surgeon are disappearing. Out here it's practically all war surgery which is so far away from civilian work. There is no cancer, none of the ordinary practice and it is only by doing that optimally that one can be good. One misses the academic side, and so much is forgotten – it is quite impossible to keep up to date with theory unless all the time one has the great incentive of teaching.

Nevertheless, entering a new year and just looking back, I'm pleased, ever so pleased that I joined the RAMC I think without patting myself on the back or anything like that, I have been of value to many wounded service men, that I have saved lives and that is sufficient satisfaction to account for any future loss whatever that may be.

Love from Stanley

The New Year came, its promise soon marred by ill news. In the Far East, the Japanese were rushing down the impassable Malay Peninsula at an incredible speed. The bloody banner of the rising sun was being carried across Burma to the very fringes of India, while at sea two of our greatest battleships had been sunk in the same action.

In Europe, the German armies were pouring into Russia. As a glimmer of hope, the early weeks of the year brought news of a new British offensive in the desert. After hold-ups and disappointments, the line was pushed beyond Sollum, leaving only remnants of the enemy in the pocket of Halfaya Pass to be subsequently winkled out from the many dugouts hewn out of the sides of its wadis. The British pressed on in a desperate endeavour to relieve Tobruk. Bardia, with its mainly Italian garrison, was cut off and surrendered and eventually the armies breaking out from the beleaguered town joined up with those of the forces beating westwards.

From the patients coming back to the hospital, we gleaned news, and casting aside the parts that disappointed, we clung hopefully to the bits that encouraged and cheered. At first it seemed that the link that joined Tobruk to the outside world was precarious, but as the prolonged battle progressed, the enemy gave ground and eventually the relief of the town was fully accomplished.

Rommel's Afrika Korps had broken off the fight and retired to its lair somewhere behind a line between Derna and Benghazi. It wasn't a beaten army, only mauled and wounded, requiring just a little time before once again it could rampage menacingly through the desert. The British Army too required time to build up stores along its attenuated lines of communication, to repair its damaged vehicles and tanks, and replace its losses before it was again ready to strike. It was a race between two armies, feverishly rebuilding their strength and recovering from their wounds, and it was to be the Afrika Korps who were ready first.

★   ★   ★

In this period of lull I was told by my CO that I was to take a few days leave, and I decided to go, with a naval friend of mine, to the Upper Nile to visit Luxor and Thebes where thousands of years before Egyptian civilisation had flourished. We arrived as short twilight turned to night and wandered quietly among the temples. The moonlight poured eerily between enormous columns and the gigantic figures of fabled gods and kings. They seemed to come to life and bewitch with their ancient power. How easy it must have been in an age when so little could be explained to believe that these figures had power over life and death, that they controlled the destiny of all men. Somewhere in these temples perhaps Moses had learned the wisdom that was to make him the leader of a great nation. Whether he was the true son of Pharaoh's daughter or not – the family of the priest Reuel believed him to be an Egyptian – he would have been brought up by the priests who were of royal blood. He would have learned the secrets of their arcane civilisation and was ready, with the authority of a God, who said, 'I am that I am', to put it to the use of another people when he fled before the wrath of Pharaoh.

A felucca with a lateen sail ferried us across the Nile when we went to see the tomb of Tutankhamun. We shared it with some fellahin and their donkeys, goats and sheep. From the ferry we mounted two of the donkeys, sitting far back on their rumps, and rode along the track which leads to the entrance of the tomb. Almost in awe we went down the very steps which, when Lord Carnarvon and Howard Carter had almost abandoned hope of finding the tomb, were famously exposed. We could feel the excitement of that fantastic discovery of two decades earlier. The steps led down into various antechambers and then into that containing the sarcophagus. The walls were painted with line upon line of figures and chariots, of gods and kings and beasts, and of scenes of conquest in ochre and brick red, black and faded white. Over a thousand years before Christ's birth, this tomb had been prepared and a World War had brought us to see it.

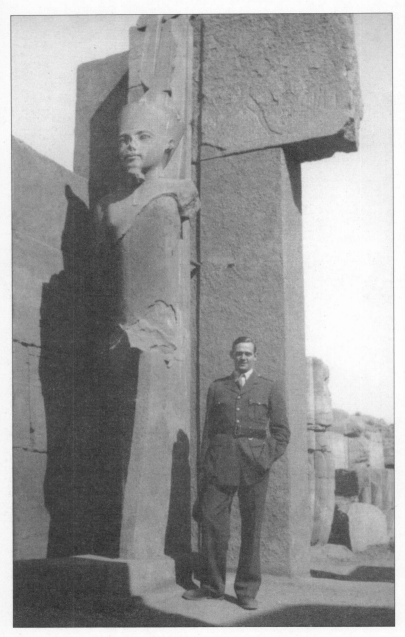

On leave in Luxor.

ON LEAVING CAIRO

I am very glad to be away from the place. Once more the nostalgia that sickens is gradually disappearing. It is not the inevitable smells: it is not the perpetual baksheesh: it is not the continual fly-whisks and dirty pictures - no, one tolerates all these - one begins to think of them as part of Egypt. It is the sickening complacency that pervades the place and disheartens one's faith in a war effort. It is the sight of staff cars coming and going and delivering their one-man burden. At the Continental, at Shepheards, at blocks of flats they roll up; and still the cry goes up: "stop this waste!"

It is the knowledge that there is an army of Base Officers in Cairo, and one knows that they are essential, but - and aye, there's the rub - is there one iota of attempt to cut down the continual expenditure and wastage? In England they cry forth for the widow's mite to build a Spitfire, and the widow's mite comes so carefully and conscientiously saved.
They say:"If you can't fight with him, fight behind him" - but is it being done in that city of glittering uniforms? Where is that sweat and toil and tears that are to be the conditions of victory? I do not see it at the Continental, at Shepheards, or at the Continental I only see the sweat of heat, the toil of peace, the tears of laughter.

How can they be making that maximum of effort with allowances of the highest order? England cries out for each penny - her need is so dire: yet a Major may be drawing up to £35 in additional pay and allowances, and spend on his actual living some £15: his pay he need not touch - that can be reserved for banking up against the day when the war ends. Blood is being spilled each minute of the day. Surely this Judas money should be stopped.

In Crete I had a friend. He was killed. His widow is given £120 by a government that can afford to pay more than three times that amount in non-taxable allowances to an Officer as cited above. It MUST be stopped if we are to win this war.

Let not this article be without construction. Let all allowances and additional pay, save for those living in hardship or in danger , be abolished for the duration of the war. Let all reasonable bills hether for messes or for living out, concerned with actual living expenses, submitted to a unit paymaster for settlement. Let us abolish allowances at allow an officer to live, drink and smoke and have without the necessity-- essity to touch his basic salary. It is the least that we can do. This war is grave, and only self-sacrifice will win it for us. THE MOMENT THE SACRIFICE IS NOT ENOUGH.

(Sgd.) STANLEY O. AYLETT.

Major, R.A.M.C.

My father's article criticises the resources wasted in support of officers' lifestyles in Cairo. It was submitted to an internal hospital paper but rejected by the editors on grounds that its contents might have a demoralising effect. Following my father's indignant response the question of expenses was eventually referred to the commanding officer.

Editorial Office,
"D" Block,
N° 64 General Hospital.

7 - 3 - 1942

Dear Major Aylett,

In many ways we agree with the views expressed in your article "On Leaving Cairo", but we feel that it is not qite in accord with the policy of this magazine.

Our policy is to provide amusement and matters of topical interest for personnel and patients of this Hospital. We feel that our rather limited public would be unable to distinguish the views you express and an attitude of defeat and despondency. Further, the reader might well think:"If these conditions really exist, why should we make any effort?"

We would suggest that your article be forwarded to an official publication which originates from G.H.Q. Such a one would be either "World Press Review" or "Gen". These publications would, of course, require your full signature but would publish your article under a nom-de-plume if so required.

If you so desire, we would be pleased to forward your article with a covering letter.

                    (Sgd.)   M.V.H. DENTON , Capt.)
                                E.L. FAWSSETT, Capt.) EDITORS--

Officers' Mess
N° 64 GENERAL HOSPITAL
M.E.F.

18 - 3 - 1942

Dear Mr. Editors,

I thank you very much for bringing my article to the notice of the Commanding Officer. It seems now that we will have achieved one slip forward towards the economies that we so loudly en–couraged and yet so poorly practised.

In my last letter with reference to the allowances at N°8 General Hospital my informant was a senior Major of the Mess. I imagine however that when he spoke of field allowancee he was probably meaning unfurnished quarters allowance and I would be pleased if you would substitute that phrase in my correspondence. The argument against it being allowable in time of war is however still as strong as ever.

You ask me whether you may copy our correspondence, and for my side I give you full permission to use it and this letter in any way in which you may consider helpful. I mention specifically this letter because I wish to quote you one example in which a few concrete figures may be given.

MY friend at N° 9 General Hospital draws additional pay allowances of £ 35-36. He pays to live at a good Pension at Heliopolis £15 a month - the price has recently been increased from £14. There is a bar in the Hospital at which drinks are purchaseable at usual mess prices so that the argument that drinks are more expensive in a hotel cuts no ice. He therefore is paid in my opinion to excess £ 20 a month. The hospital has some 26 officers. All are not drawing such heavy allowances. Let us assume that on an average allowances are £ 25 and this, I would, I am sure be below the actual figure. That mess is therefore overpaid about £ 2600 a year for the privilege of living in comparative luxury in Cairo. This is just one mess, - just 26 officers.

To conclude I would be pleased if you would be kind enough to let me have copy of our correspondence and my article.

Yours faithfully,

STANLEY O. AYLETT.

Major, R.A.M.C.

11

DEPARTURE FOR
THE DESERT

MARCH–MAY 1942

*Attached to an Indian casualty clearing station
along the coast before being posted to Tobruk*

On my return from leave I asked to see the CO. I had been
with the hospital for a year and I wanted, once again, to
see if it was possible to work in forward units. I had heard that a
surgical team was to be sent from No. 64 to join desert units and
I asked him if when this team was formed I could be considered
as its surgeon. While having some rather nice things to say about
me, he told me that he would not stand in my way and certainly I
could go. Very soon after, I was summoned to the colonel's office
and told that I would be leaving in a few days, that I was to select
another officer to go with me, as well as two nursing orderlies, and
that we would be attached to an Indian casualty clearing station
where we would be joined by an anaesthetist from that unit.

I had no difficulty in finding my three colleagues. I chose for my officer Captain Ian MacIver. I knew that he was a first-class doctor and, if called upon, he was a competent anaesthetist and a surgeon as well. As important was the fact that he was an imperturbable and charming person with a tenor voice with which he could entertain us at the drop of a hat. He came from Newcastle, and there had acted in and produced operas and plays. Naturally he had been in charge of the drama section of our social activities at the hospital. On one occasion, in a review, he had contrived a sketch consisting of two very brief acts. The first was: 'The officers' mess as other ranks believe it to be'. The curtain went up on a scene of some debauchery, with semi-drunken officers lounging about the place or entertaining nurses on sofas in the most compromising of positions. The curtain fell. The next act was: 'The officers' mess as it actually is', and the curtain went up on precisely the same scene. The unit and the patients loved it.

The night before we left, Ian and I were given a magnificent party and our heads were perhaps not entirely clear as we loaded the three-tonner. We left our hospital with mixed feelings. It was a wrench to say goodbye to such grand colleagues as we had had, and we were sad to be leaving not only one of the best of hospitals but one that had been for us a very happy home. On the other hand we were glad because we felt that the war was soon to move far away and that we were following it to do the job for which we had joined the army – the early surgical treatment of wounded troops. Not for one moment did it cross our minds that before many months had passed we should be back again.

We took with us a reasonable amount of stores and surgical equipment but we had no tents or surgical beds and no transport of our own. The field surgical unit, self-contained and complete, had still not been finally evolved and our unit now was little more than the surgical team of BEF days.

The road westwards runs out from Alexandria along the coast.

The fringes of the town are lined with smallholdings where, by dint of hard work on the part of the farmers, somehow the poor sandy soil is induced to yield a crop of wheat or maize. Farther out still there are groves of fig trees, tended by groups of desert wanderers, living very close to the earth in the squalor of their torn and tattered tents, where the fowls are as much at home as the children crawling about their floors. Beyond these groves the desert road stretches mile upon mile into the distance. Here and there, where it nears the coast, the monotony of the drab landscape is relieved by patches of scrub grass, brightened with purple and gold rock flowers in the early springtime. Now and then you pass a line of camels plodding the long miles slowly away, their owners oblivious to the war that stranger nations have brought to their familiar desert. Only army transport, tanks, guns and lorries roar up and down this highway.

Nearly a hundred miles from Alexandria is Mersa Matruh, a small town built round an azure blue lagoon. Before the war it had been a holiday resort for the cities of Egypt, with large hotels and weekend villas. Now it was only a skeleton town of roofless houses, scarred and pitted by war, with its lagoon disfigured by barbed wire and rusted vehicles.

At Mersa was a line-of-communication unit of the RAMC and like so many of its kind, it neither possessed the cool efficiency of a base unit nor the enthusiasm of a forward one. All it wished for was to be left alone in peace and quiet, and visitors of a junior rank, even though they were reporting in accordance with instructions, were left in no doubt that they were a nuisance, disturbing a humdrum routine that no doubt included an afternoon siesta. After several hours' wait, during which time we cast envious eyes on the cups of tea that passed in and out of this inhospitable office, we were informed that we were to proceed to our Indian casualty clearing station the following day, spending the night here at a local transit camp.

We arrived next afternoon and reported to the commanding officer of the CCS who, not surprisingly, had had no warning of our arrival. But this was a forward unit which had seen service in both the Abyssinian and desert campaigns, and hospitality was not only given, but given very gladly to any visitors.

On and off we worked for several weeks in this unit and each day increased the regard with which we viewed our CO. Each Indian unit was staffed partly by British, partly by Eurasians and partly by Indians, the latter including Hindus, Muslims and Untouchables, and all had to be welded together so that all their separate differences were strictly subordinate to the main purpose of the CCS. It was not easy to run an efficient unit with such initial difficulties, but somehow these were lost in the charm and personality of the CO.

It would be idle to pretend that the unit was as good as a British CCS. The Indian orderlies had little of the basic education upon which to build an elementary standard of nursing or of medicine and surgery, and with few exceptions the Indian medical officers were not of the same professional standard as their European colleagues. This war to them was something apparently remote from Indian interests and because of that they did not bring with them the enthusiasm, without which a really hard slog is impossible. Many of them saw it as another aberration of an imperialistic Raj, but they had been tempted into the service by the very high rates of pay, three or four times as much as that which they were likely to earn back home. That these differences of opinion were so submerged, and that a fairly united and reasonably happy unit did exist, all depended on the personality of the CO who, ignoring the differences, concentrated on the similarities. When, I thought, India gained independence and men like this were given their discharge from the Indian Medical Service, the losers would be India and Indian medicine.

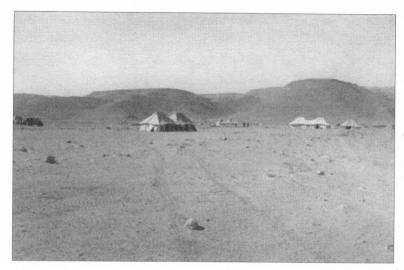

Desert camp.

This CCS was set up in the plain of sand that lies between Sollum and Halfaya, bounded behind by a steep escarpment and in front by the blue sea. Casualties in this waiting period were few, but each day there were the unfortunates who had trodden on a hidden mine or booby trap, or those who, with misplaced inquisitiveness, had picked up a detonator or some disguised explosive with disastrous results. We learned very quickly that before one picked up anything in this area of desert, extreme wariness was necessary as the enemy had been there for a long time and had had ample opportunity to set its traps.

Along the road that bordered the sea a constant stream of transport, growing heavier each day, was travelling west beyond Sollum towards the front. Guns and tank transporters with their huge burdens rattled noisily along and somehow navigated the steep hairpin bends of the pass that led up to the top of the escarpment.

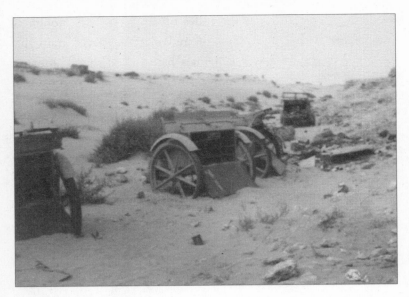

Mussolini's desert debris.

We were waiting, hoping each day would bring news of the great battle for which preparations were so obviously being pushed forward. But although we waited many weeks, it was not a time that from our point of view was wasted, because we were novices in the desert and we had to learn how to live and work in these very different conditions.

Above all else we had to learn the value of water. Neither of us was new to forward surgery, as we had served in Belgium and France when conditions, to say the least, were difficult. But we had always had ample supplies of water to drink, to wash in and to do all the sterilisation and cleaning necessary in an operating theatre. Now, literally, every cupful was of value. Deeper in the desert, engineers were busy extending the pipeline that was to carry thousands of gallons of water from hundreds of miles away in Alexandria far up beyond Sollum. On water the whole life of the army depended. True, there were numerous natural water points scattered through the miles of sand, but not enough to supply the demands of machine and man. Even the train that chugged along its newly laid lines had a thirst on its journey equivalent to that of thousands of men. For success, water was as essential as petrol and oil, and as such it was guarded as jealously as these other fluids.

On the coast we were miles from the water line and drew our supplies from two natural wells. The brackish water, so salted that you drank it from necessity and not for pleasure, was rigorously rationed. We learned that it was quite possible to go through all early-morning ablutions on a large mugful of water. There was a routine that had to be followed, but at least you were left with the feeling that you had washed. First you cleaned your teeth and then proceeded to shave, taking care not to wash your razor in the mug. Then, with the aid of sponge or flannel dampened with what remained, you had a rub-down. If not complete, your wash was at least refreshing.

This lack of a sufficient quantity of water for washing purposes may have had something to do with the sores that broke out among troops who had been stationed in the desert for months on end. They were constantly covered with the dry desert dust, which readily adhered to bodies always moist in the heat. It was rarely possible to get really clean, and small cuts and abrasions, which on a normally clean skin would have healed rapidly, became infected and spread to form large ulcers. They were peculiar to the desert, these sores, and were hardly ever seen among base troops where washing facilities were always available.

It was in the operating theatre particularly that economy had to be exercised. Without thoughtful and vigilant care, enormous quantities could be consumed very readily. There were the bowls of water in which the surgeon and his assistant had to scrub their hands. More was required in which to sterilise instruments and to clean up the patient before his operation. Lotions had to be made up and, above all, at the end of an operating session there was laundering to be done so that blood-stained towels would be clean and ready for sterilisation once again. It was obvious that without economy our rations would rapidly run out if there were a large number of casualties, and in order to avoid this we recycled the used water by filtering it through sand. Water in any medical unit in the desert was always an underlying worry. If you had an extra forty gallons or so tucked away in your lorry, you were that much happier about any difficulties of supply that might arise.

So the time passed and we waited, learning each day some new idea by means of which a desert operating theatre could be improved and preparing our stores and dressings for the battle we knew was imminent. In addition, we were becoming familiar with desert life, and finding by experiment and error how best one could live in reasonable comfort. We were learning that even in summer the sun does not always shine but can be blotted out for days on end by a sandstorm more impenetrable than a London fog; even during the day you could get hopelessly lost over the shortest journey. We were learning, too, that in spite of its monotony, the desert had its beauty, especially when the sun rose red as fire or sank flaming into the sea.

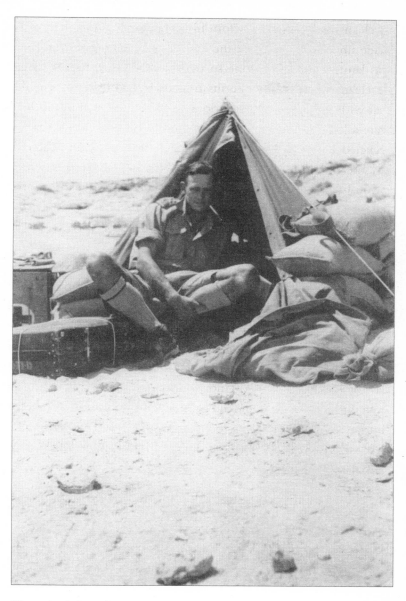

The author's desert home.

I wrote three letters home from this CCS.

Sunday, 19 April 1942
Major S. O. Aylett, RAMC
No. 2 Indian CCS, MEF

My dear Mum and Dad – The above is as you see my new address but as it is unlikely to be very permanent, for the present I should address any letters to No. 64 and they will send them on wherever we may be.

We are camped in the desert fairly close to the sea in one of the most fought over areas of this war. All around are the relics of defeated armies. There are guns and lorries, tanks and armoured cars, all now a mass of twisted and deformed metal. Here and there are little collections of crosses to show the cost that this little area of sand has extracted. Some have inscriptions in English, some in German and others in Italian. Wherever you look there are shell cases, empty tins and discarded rifles and hand grenades, tin hats often riddled with bullet holes, clothing, gas masks, bandoliers, all in one awful confusion. The north of France must have looked like this when we left, except that here it is dull hardened desert instead of green fields.

Behind us a range of hills towers up, honeycombed with little holes in which men have lived like animals to escape the mass of high explosive poured upon them. Here in these hills, too, can be found all the debris and scars of war.

A few miles away are some ruins which once were a town by the sea. Nothing remains except rubble and stones and guns and twisted burned-out vehicles. Inscriptions on the remaining walls tell that sometimes this town was in Italian hands and sometimes in British.

And now I suppose we wait here for the next battle, which will produce another patch of desert to equal this. I am very glad to be here. I have two excellent lads with me as well as my fellow officer. I am feeling very ready and fit for hard work and I think that if it comes we will make a good show of it.

My love to you both,
Stanley

8 May 1942
Major S. O. Aylett
No. 2 Mobile Surgical Team, MEF

My dear Mum and Dad – In the last few days a dust storm has raged. This is a gale blowing about 50 to 60 miles an hour off the desert, filled with grit and sand. It blows first from the south so that everywhere it is like a hot oven, and then from the north, when it approaches an icy blast. It's just like a fickle woman, but always grit and sand which hits and stings. The visibility yesterday at midday was less than in a London fog of the worst type and you could not see 10 yards in front of you. It's simplicity itself to lose one's way simply walking from one tent to another. Sand lies about an inch deep on everything – it collects as fast as you can shake it away, so it's no use trying to get rid of it until it stops blowing. It clings to clothes and hair and skin until you look like a pillar of sand. Is this what happened to Lot's wife? Only when too much collects in your eyes – because it manages to find its way through any goggles which one has to wear – do you rub it out? The other night, to add to the confusion of the sandstorm, our tent blew down so that there was a period of indescribable chaos when everything seemed to have got mixed up with everything else. What food or drink we have is served with sand. You can understand what they mean on the wireless when they say 'dust storms held up operations'.

So far, the bombs have all been nicely distant and not too frequent. You know, the sort of distance away when you can go out and have a look at the fireworks and say, 'Well I'm glad I'm not one of those poor buggers over there.' Today we will sort out the dust, as this morning has started off peacefully and filled with sunshine.

I'm glad to be here. One appreciates now what our troops have to put up with. I prefer being a desert rat to a base wallah. We have not been very busy but I have done about a dozen major ops, with, I think, success, so we are justifying our existence.

My love to you,

Stanley

May 18 No. 2 Mobile Surgical Unit/No. 20 Indian Field Ambulance

We have left the Field Ambulance and are back in our Indian CCS...

We still await the real thing. Life in the army it has been said consists of periods of intense boredom doing little, and of times of great excitement when you've much too much to do. When the time comes life will be very difficult because surgery in what at present constitutes the so-called mobile unit is far from easy. There's the ever-present sand blowing up into storms to contend with. There are difficulties in lighting, difficulties in sterilisation and a host of other problems.

They could all be solved so easily if only we had a mobile theatre on wheels. But they (the powers that be) seem only to have just thought how essential it is and I suppose that in another year's time I should have one. They are so simple to plan and arrange. I remember when we came back from France. I and a pal had line drawings made of one. That was 2 years ago, and when submitted it was looked on with extreme disfavour. I don't think the younger generation had much to do with the making of this war, and I doubt whether they will have much to do with the actual fashioning of it, except to cheerfully die in it...

The light is getting low and the sun is setting which is probably as well else I should develop on a theme I feel very bitter about. I know youthful ideas cannot do everything but they can do a lot better than many old ones, but they are not allowed.

Love from Stanley

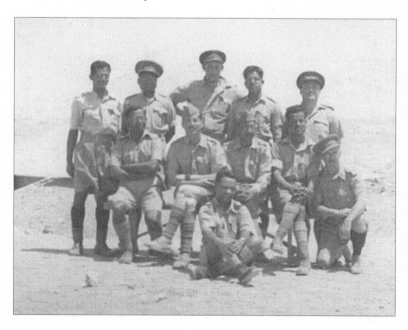

The author (centre, back row) while attached to an Indian CCS.

In the evenings before supper the colonel and ourselves eked out a very small supply of whisky, diluting it freely with the salted water because that was the only way to make it last. Fortunately, only one or two of the Indian officers took alcohol. Somehow the unit's cook transformed the ordinary army rations, adding spices and curries, and always there were chapattis.

The CO had spent most of his life in India and countries in the East, and entertained us over supper with his stories. He told us of a murderer who would never be convicted of his crime. He, the colonel, had been sent as surgeon to a British Embassy in one of the countries bordering India. A mixed collection of representatives of many European nations, mainly men, lived in the capital – diplomatic staffs, merchants, engineers and other technicians – and naturally, as they were few in number, they saw a good deal of each other. It was soon obvious that the stage was set for tragedy and drama.

Each night the younger men of the small station gathered around a beautiful German girl – the wife of a businessman much older than herself – in admiration of her charm and of her personality, and one in particular fell desperately in love. Wherever a party was held he would be, standing nearby or, if fortune favoured him, sitting by her side with all his feelings written plainly over his face. The girl grew more lovely and playful in this sunshine of passion and admiration, but jealousy and hate smouldered in the older man who was her husband. Now and then his temper flared out beyond control and only the calming words of other members of the colony prevented ugly scenes.

One evening, the German and his wife gave a dinner party in their house. The night was humid and hot. To all who were present it was obvious that bitter words had passed between husband and wife. The guests talked together, ill at ease and restrained. They knew somehow that tonight was filled with danger and yet it seemed inevitable and unpreventable. There was nothing they could do.

The German was drinking more heavily than usual. On a settee his wife sat talking with her friend as if defying circumstances and fate. Suddenly the storm broke. The German rushed towards his wife and seized her by her shoulders. 'I will kill you,' he shouted, 'if ever I see you making love to this man again.'

His friends tried to restrain and calm him, and his wife, bursting into tears, fled out of the room and rushed upstairs. They heard the key of her bedroom door turn in the lock. Her husband broke away from his friends and followed his wife. They heard him hammering on the door demanding to be let in, and then a crash as the door gave way. As they stood there wondering what to do, revolver shots rang out. They rushed upstairs, and through the broken door saw the German bent weeping over the unconscious figure of his wife.

She was taken to hospital but in spite of immediate surgery she died. Whatever the provocation and intention, this was murder, and as such should have been tried by the law of the country in which it was committed. But all, and especially the German legation, realised that the prestige of the European colony would suffer untold harm if such a trial were held in a native court. It was therefore agreed that the German should be sent home through India under the protection of the British authorities and that his wife's death should be attributed to an accident. When he arrived home the charges against him would be presented in his own country.

Accordingly, he was sent down through India to Bombay to be embarked on a British ship sailing to Europe. The year was 1939, the month August. With war imminent, the ship's sailing was postponed. On 3 September, Herr Schmidt was removed for internment. No murder charge had yet been presented against him, and from a country at war with England it never would be. The outbreak of hostilities had saved his life.

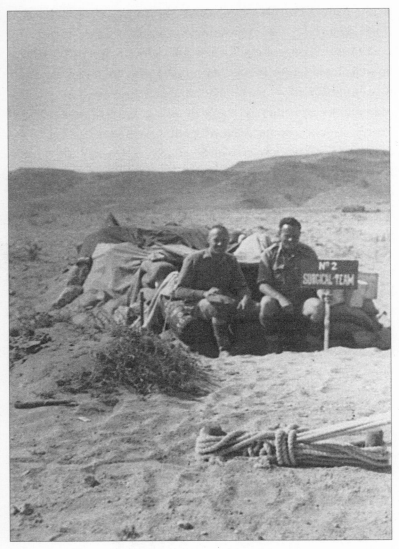

Desert homes of officers and orderlies, No. 2 Surgical Team.

★   ★   ★

At the end of May, Rommel's Afrika Korps roared out of its lair. It had won the race of preparation and again held the initiative. In spite of that, however, confidence ran high that shortly we would be well on the way to Tripoli. My surgical team was at once ordered to Tobruk and we were to be accompanied by one of the Indian anaesthetists from the CCS as well as his bearer. Our tents were rapidly taken down and along with our equipment were loaded on to one of the unit's lorries, which was to take us as far as Capuzzo. As we left our site and joined the coast road we could see in the distance Halfaya Pass, which led from the end of the bay up to the top of the escarpment. It was obscured by a haze of dusty sand thrown up by the hundreds and hundreds of vehicles and tanks and guns which were already climbing its crudely surfaced zig-zag road. Driving over the challenging surfaces of desert track was no light job for the RASC drivers.

At the top of the pass several streams of vehicles converged, so that almost nose to tail, reinforcements of all descriptions were pouring up towards the battlefront. Everywhere there was an atmosphere of relief. All the tension of the long days of waiting had suddenly abated. The army was once more to measure its strength against the Afrika Korps and there was hopeful confidence in the result. True those guns pushing out of the turrets of the tanks looked terribly small: you did not want to look at them too long because they left you feeling uncomfortable. You had heard the enemy had 88mm guns and these two-pounders, you felt, were puny by comparison. The tank crews looked sunburned and confident, clinging to their iron castles as they lurched unsteadily along. Perhaps they, too, had doubts, but if they had they did not show. Speaking to them earlier, they had now and again gazed longingly at those barrels as if the ideal they saw in their imaginations might suddenly sprout from these small versions. But this was all they had now, and they were going to make the best of it.

Not far from the top of the escarpment lies Fort Capuzzo, outpost of Mussolini's Libyan empire, now devastated by bombardment from the air and land and from the sea; only a broken eagle and sceptre lying awry on its side remained to remind one of the grandiose ambitions of a dictator. Close by was a cemetery, one of so many scattered along the desert tracks where armies had fought and passed. It was not simple and restful like our own because swastika and iron-cross emblems with their twisted and garbled messages had been chosen to mark the graves of their dead. It was to all appearances, a pagan resting ground, aggressive and abrasive even in death.

From Capuzzo we were driven by American drivers who belonged to a volunteer corps which had for months been driving ambulances up and down the desert. They had volunteered for medical service with the British Army long before America entered the war (in December 1941). Their members came from all walks of life. Some were medical students, some solicitors, others artisans and tradesmen. If you asked them why they had left their homes when the USA was still at peace, all might have replied as one did to me, 'Oh well, we thought you might have been in kind of a jam and we wanted to come and help.' It was thrilling to think that all the might of another nation was now fighting with us and grand to have such audible evidence of it by one's side.

I have never been so frightened on any journey as on that trip up to Tobruk. I arrived sweating gently, not only from the heat of the summer's day but from sheer terror. My American driver told me he was going to drive fast, his explanation being a very simple and reasonable one, to him. 'It's like this, doc,' he said. 'I've been back late on the last two nights and when you get back late the food is ruined, so I'll be gawddamned damned if I'll be back late tonight because I want my evening meal.' He passed every vehicle that came in sight. It did not matter whether the road narrowed so that he had to go off on to the dangerously soft sand on the verges. It did not matter if the visibility was reduced to a few yards by the clouds of dust set up by a thousand vehicles. It was all the same – the accelerator was on the floorboard. Twice vehicles in front of us toppled over as they ran off the road into the sand. For a few brief seconds his foot then came off the accelerator and his head went out of the window to shout, 'Are you OK?' to the drivers scrambling out of their cabs, then away he went again. Most of the time he was driving one-handed as he was covered in the rash of scabies and required one hand to scratch away vigorously at the various points of acute irritation. I tactfully pointed out to him that he had this complaint, picked up no doubt from some dirty blanket, and the sooner he had it treated so much the better for himself and his comrades. 'Gee, doc, is that scabies?' he said. 'And the boys said I'd just got a bit of a sweat rash. I'll sure come and see you in Tobruk.' He came and the scabies soon disappeared.

All the gods who look after travellers on the Tobruk road must have been guarding us that evening because as the sun was settling on the sea, we came towards the town. As we rounded the last curve of the road before it started to descend, we could see Tobruk half a mile or so away. It all looked so lovely and innocent from the distance with its little white houses built on the side of a hill. Some of them seemed reddened as they reflected the light of the dying sun. What we could not see from afar was that not one of those houses was complete, that all were battered and scarred by bullets and bombardment. We could not see that so many of the ships – scores of them – that seemed to be peacefully at anchor in the blue harbour were in fact lying quietly on the seabed. Only when you were close was illusion dispelled.

12

THE MOVE TO TOBRUK

MAY–JUNE 1942

Conditions in the Tobruk hospital; retreat with the
Eighth Army; return to No. 64 General Hospital, Alexandria

The hospital was set up in what had been the Italian barracks.
It consisted of a series of modern buildings that, although
some had been bombed and damaged during the siege, still
provided reasonable accommodation.

The RAMC is relatively small in any command and it is seldom
you move to a new unit without meeting friends with whom you
have worked before, and here in Tobruk were many. It is better that
way because working in association with colleagues you know the
routine at once runs along smooth and easy lines. A great friend
of mine, Colonel Simpson Smith, to whom I have referred before,
was in charge of the surgical side of the hospital. He was one of
those people who are completely tireless. No matter how hard
he worked in the operating theatres – and he worked equal shifts

with all of us – there was not a patient who left the hospital to go on the evacuating ambulances that he did not first visit in order to make quite sure they were comfortable and fit enough to cope with the journey that lay ahead. Day after day, until just before the fall of the town, his routine went on. In spite of it all, in spite of the fact that in each twenty-four-hour period his sleeping hours could have been counted on the four fingers of one hand, he remained charming and debonair, enthusiastic for any improvement that could be made, steadfastly sympathetic and kind in the face of all the suffering in that hospital.

I think he must have had a presentiment that one day he would be captured. Down in the Canal Zone his conversation would often turn to means of escaping. He studied maps, read books of escape, worked out various possibilities suitable for different circumstances, planned and to an extent practised them. At that time, when we were together, we agreed that if ever that evil day came, we should somehow make a break for it. Fortune found me away from Tobruk when it finally came. SS, as he was affectionately known to all, was captured. He made a gallant effort to get away – and was never seen again. Somewhere in the sands around Tobruk he rests, close to the hospital where he had done work more exacting than any asked of him in the quiet nursing homes around Harley Street in which he practised before the war.

Soon after our arrival, the casualties starting pouring in and the wounded lay everywhere. On stretcher stands, on beds, on the floor, head to toe and toe to head. Smashed-in faces, shattered limbs, guts wrecked by high explosive, chests into which God's fresh air can no longer be drawn – they had every injury imaginable. At one end of the main reception ward there was a screened-off section. There we had to put those who, grossly wounded, seem likely to die. They were barely conscious. They didn't know why they were being separated from their comrades. But in spite of the fact that most of these

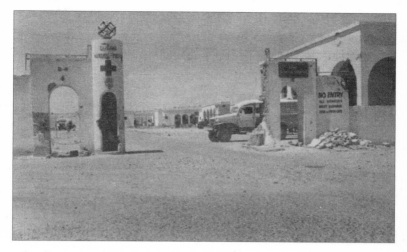

Italian barracks were used as a hospital in Tobruk.

wounded didn't stand a chance, we did not give up. There were a few who might regain the precious life that was all but lost once we got new blood slowly dripping back into their veins.

Now and then an orderly came and covered up a face. I did not know why they covered up their faces when they die, but I suppose it was in the rules. Admittedly death is not a pretty sight and its serenity a fiction, but they did not look any better when they were so desperately close to life's end. Compared to that perhaps they did look at peace.

There seemed to be a lot of padres about. Every so often one threw a coloured band about his neck and administered the last rites. This seemed to sanctify death, perhaps make it all a little less horrible.

We operated in a long room. There were eight tables with doctors hard at work and a continual to and fro of patients being lifted on and lifted off. At first the room was clean and orderly, but it rapidly deteriorated. There was blood and carved-off flesh on the floor, dirty dressings and white splashes of plaster of Paris.

There was little water and little time to clear it all up except when it became really impossible. The bowls in which you washed your hands got steadily dirtier in spite of filtering the water. Water was so precious and there was not nearly enough of it.

Everyone was sweating profusely. There was no ventilation and the blackout was rigidly enforced. The night is hot and the Primus sterilisers added their heat to make it worse. Now and then one of them flared up, sending a shower of sooty flakes to blacken the faces of all who were working nearby. There was none of the quiet hush of a theatre at home. Instead there were the excited screams and curses and oaths of men who fought the pain as the anaesthetic was poured on. We were in very short supply of the anaesthetic Pentothal, which puts a man to sleep most quietly and rapidly, as a large consignment had recently been sunk on its way out from England; so we had to use older methods.

My anaesthetist was an Indian. In some ways I thought that he talked the patients to sleep, leaning over them, stroking their foreheads with soothing hands and calming them with a droning voice. He was very good but his only trouble was that every four hours or so he decided he has had enough and needed a rest. I plead with him, cajole and curse him, and point out that many of the waiting wounded are his own people, but it made no difference and off he went to some corner where his Untouchable bearer will make him comfortable and bring him food. My other officer, Captain MacIver, then, instead of helping me, had to give the anaesthesia, and one of my orderlies act as my assistant. After a couple of hours my Indian friend returned refreshed, to continue his very good work but we were not on the best of terms.

Now and then there was a rush to a table of all available hands, where a soldier in the first stages of anaesthesia had suddenly gone fighting mad. He is forced down, more dope was poured on and his struggles slowly subsided, while his words became incoherent and sobbing. Comparative peace descended again.

Then there were the calls of, 'Stretcher bearers', 'Catgut, please', 'Spencer Wells', 'Vomit dish, quick', while the atmosphere became steadily worse, until you had to go away for a few moments to breathe in some cool fresh air.

Outside an air raid was going on. Machine guns tapped viciously; there was the scream and roar of a diving plane. Even as you continued with the operation there is a part of you that is waiting for it to unload. Suddenly there was a God-almighty crash and the few remaining panes of the window came tinkling in. But until the next time it was over for now, and you could give your whole and undivided attention to the operation, although your heart would be beating a little faster.

The work went on. The torn bodies were patched up. The dead and dying tissue was cut away, limbs smashed beyond the broad margin of repair and recovery were amputated. In so far as was possible, we tried to maintain the principles of aseptic surgery, but from that ideal, so easy in a peacetime operating theatre at home, we can't help falling short. We knew that if we did not attain that ideal, wounds would go septic, prolonging the period of recovery, even now and then producing a fatal result.

But with water so short, with time so limited, with conditions far from good, we could do nothing more than try our hardest and our best. Sometimes we thought there was no chance and yet we operated. Now and then we pulled back someone from the brink, someone who was probably everything in the world to an unknown person a thousand and more miles away, and we had an indescribable feeling of thankfulness that a life had been saved. There was no feeling of self-satisfaction, none of the, 'I'm a good surgeon, look what I've done'. No, it was just the thrill of turning the tables on death. It was the thrill of seeing the purity of life returning instead of the stench and filth of wounds and death.

We had two small side theatres. These we reserved only for those soldiers with wounds to the abdomen or to the chest or head. In these little rooms there was still fresh and clean water and there were operating gowns and gloves, so that as far as possible we could operate under reasonably sterile conditions. Here we sewed up holes in the intestine, cut away too badly damaged sections and joined the ends together, remove lacerated kidneys and spleens torn asunder by shells and explosives, and sutured vast rents in the liver. We picked out the spicules of bone and metal driven into the brain and repaired large holes in the chest, and we breathed a prayer to God to let them recover. They looked clean and comfortable, these wounded, as they were carried off the operating table in their nice white bandages. That dull red ooze had not yet soaked through the gauze and cotton wool and they were at peace too, in anaesthetic unconsciousness, but the journey to recovery had only just begun.

There were two marvellous sisters in this theatre block. Whatever the difficulties or the troubles, they were there helping us and the wounded to bear up, and working as hard as anyone.

We looked forward to the dawn. Then we knew the racket of air raids would die down and we could pull the blackout curtains apart and let the fresh air blow in through the glassless window. We knew that the steady stream of ambulances that had been coming in all night would tail off. It was difficult to move the wounded down from the forward collecting posts during the daytime and most arrived in darkness.

Even when no more ambulances drew into the hospital there were still hours more work ahead dealing with those men who were already filling our reception ward. But you could see an end to it and a chance of getting the theatre cleaned up, visiting the patients who had survived their operations, and sleeping a little before nightfall again brought the ambulances streaming in.

★　★　★

The days and nights passed by. Optimism ran high and the lightly wounded were in high spirits with the way the battle was going. We too found things to laugh at in our few off-duty hours. We had a pig we had named Rommel, and watching his steadily increasing girth, we saw a vision of the enormous leg of pork that one day would be carried into our mess. It was not a very kind vision and one was a little embarrassed by it because Rommel was a friendly animal, wandering about with an affectionate grunt for whoever cared to pass the time of day with him. But though we did not know it, envious eyes from neighbouring units were cast on Rommel and one evening we heard the roar of an army truck and the very indignant squeals of protest from our pig who was resenting strongly the rude assault that had been made upon him.

Fortunately, he struggled hard and managed to topple over the backboard of the truck into which he had been bundled, and his kidnappers drove away rapidly, happily without our prospective dinner. In order to avoid any further risk, Rommel had to be slaughtered a little before his time.

I wrote to my parents from Tobruk.

8 June 1942
Major S. O. Aylett, RAMC
No. 2 Mobile Surgical Team, MEF

My dear Mum and Dad – If I was writing to any of my friends I could only open my letter with one phrase to explain my feelings, and as you are friends as well as parents I say, and you must forgive me, 'Christ, what a week.' We've worked flat out just snatching an hour's rest now and then. Once again we have all the awfulness of shattered bodies lying on the floor head to head with not an inch between them, waiting their turn to come to the surgeon. Limbs bent and unnatural in their brokenness, faces that look like smashed pulp, heads where the brain oozes out, the little room set aside for the dying, the stink, the filth, the flies, the absolute shambles, following a night's work, of blood and dressings and plaster and cut-off clothes.

That's briefly what being a surgeon in a forward area is like. One operates on the less injured and on the hopeless case, and now and then the hopeless case recovers. It's like a gleam of sunshine in a stormy sky. The other night I operated on six such cases. Four died – four to five hours' sweat and toil just wasted – but the fifth, stinking with gas gangrene, liable to die any minute on the operating table, is living and getting better after having his arm and shoulder taken away. The sixth lingers.

At night the bombers add confusion. The roar of a powerful barrage, that whine of falling bombs and work is our lot. Last night a stick fell in the hospital but apart from blowing out the window sashes all was well.

I am happier than for a long time now, feeling I am doing a good job of work. No longer a base wallah, but a hard-working bloke for a change.

At the minute we are in that much besieged port but I do not think it will be besieged again as this time Jerry has met his match.

Must go now,

Love from

Stanley

How wrong I was.

One day all the hope and cheerfulness that in spite of everything pervaded our work was dimmed. The survivors of tank crew after tank crew were being brought in, often cruelly burned. They told us how all seemed to have gone wrong in their attack and how they had been shelled by heavier guns without a chance of replying adequately with their small two-pounders. The victory that we had hoped for so fervently was turning into defeat. A day had changed the fortune of a battle and the old story of retreat loomed up again.

The air raids on Tobruk increased in intensity as if the enemy knew that this town, for which they had battled nearly eighteen months, was at last within their grasp. The hospital was lucky and bombs fell only on empty buildings. One large eleven-hundred-pounder buried itself in a block away from the theatre but failed to explode. When we went outside to see what had produced this louder than average whistle and crump, we were startled to see three fins projecting from a large crater.

Shellfire, which in the last few days had seemed to move away from Tobruk, was now coming obviously closer and the ambulances were coming through enemy pockets on their way to the hospital. There was an air of gloom over everything and it soon became obvious that Tobruk would not be defended for very long if it were cut off. Heavy guns and equipment were being moved out of the town and orders came for our sisters to be evacuated by a hospital ship that was leaving the harbour.

We were sad to see them go. A hospital can never be the same efficient unit without the help and skill of nursing sisters, however excellent the RAMC nursing orderlies are. They on their side had no wish to leave but it was an order and a correct one. A few days later a morning came when there was not a single patient in the hospital. We had evacuated everyone by hospital ship, and ambulances were not getting through the cordon that once again almost completely surrounded Tobruk.

My surgical team and I were ordered back to join the Eighth Army. We were chosen as we were the only unit attached to the hospital that carried full surgical operating equipment. It was those few scalpels and forceps, our dressing drums and sterilisers, which prevented us from becoming prisoners of war.

We said our goodbyes, expecting that the colleagues who we were leaving behind would be in Alexandria long before ourselves as we supposed the garrison was to be evacuated by sea. We did not expect that all would be taken prisoner and that two of our friends would be killed as a result of brave endeavours to escape

Our gear was loaded into a Friends' ambulance, one of the fleet run entirely by the Quakers, which was going eastwards. The road leaving Tobruk was being shelled and we left it to roar along the hard desert sand before rejoining it further down.

We were attached to an Indian field ambulance near Halfaya Pass and opened a theatre in a cave hewn out of the rock itself. It had been used by the Germans when it was their turn to struggle to hold this pass. It was far from ideal but at least had the merit of having a roof of several hundreds of feet of solid rock.

It soon became very evident, however, that this border of Egypt was not going to limit the retreat. Columns were pulling out of Sollum, which meant the road down towards Mersa Matruh was filled with vehicles. Had the Luftwaffe had sufficient air power it seemed that most of the Eighth Army could have been wiped out that day. But once again the RAF with its South African comrades stood between it and disaster. Forward aerodromes were being evacuated but from further back the cover was maintained.

Stage by stage we retreated. For a few hours in one place or

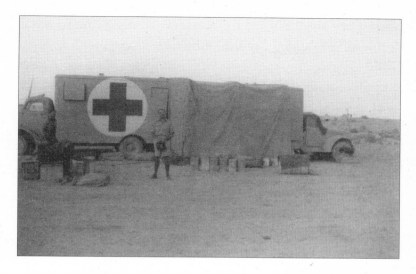

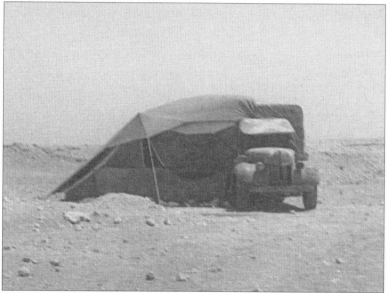

Mobile operating theatres in the desert.

another we set up our theatre, operated and packed up to repeat our work fifty miles closer to Alexandria. Sometimes we had a tent to operate in, sometimes it was just a shelter thrown out from the side of a lorry. Only the most urgent type of surgery could we tackle in these circumstances.

For a few days outside Mersa Matruh we were lucky enough to have an Egyptian barracks in which to operate, but with the enemy's rapid advance, shelling soon made it untenable and we were ordered back to No. 64 General Hospital. The battle had lasted about four weeks, but they were weeks that made the dream of Tripoli seem as remote as the end of the war itself.

SUBJECT Reports, Fd. Surgical Units.

    Maj AYLETT (No 6 M.E. Fd. Surgical Unit)

D.Q.

                                   GHQ. MEF.
                                   7.7.42

Dear *Aylett*,

      Your report (dated 29.6.42) has just arrived. I enjoyed reading it immensely, and I congratulate you not only on your good work and the soundness of your general remarks, but on your spirit. I know full well that you had many unpleasant and anxious times. The surgery, as we have seen it at the base this time, has been first rate, and there has been an all round improvement even on that of the previous battle.

      Your remarks on your assistant made me laugh. I fear you would not be a "suitable" officer for service in India ! ?   You must realise that your assistant was sent forward for necessary training in this type of work.

      I enclose a Memo. on "Surgical Teams" which, I hope, will explain much, including the absence of transport.(official)

      We have already issued a note on the terms which should be used in describing surgical procedures in connection with operations on wounds.   These agree, in essence, with your remarks.

      I hope it may be possible to relieve some of the forward surgical units, but it was considered inadvisable to embarrass Staffs (Q. Movt. etc) until the situation is a little more stabilised.   It looks, as though you would like to continue for a while.?

      I am being returned to U.K. - as you probably know - shortly, and Ogilvie takes over. May I, in conclusion, thank you for your good work and wish you good luck.

                          Yrs sincerely,

                          (D.C. Monro) Maj. Gen.
                          Consultant Surgeon MEF.

Maj. S. AYLETT RAMC.
   64 BGH-

Letter of 7 July 1942 from Major-General Monro, Consultant Surgeon MEF, acknowledging receipt of the author's final report on the work of No.2 Surgical Team.

13

THE EXODUS FROM ALEXANDRIA

JULY 1942–MAY 1943

*At the casualty clearing stations in the desert in the run-up to
the battle of El Alamein; return to Alexandria immediately before
the battle to receive casualties at No. 64 General Hospital;
rejoicing at victory; arrival of spring*

B ack in Alexandria, the news of the desert defeat had brought
gloom. It seemed both to the civilian and to the serviceman
that there was now little to prevent Rommel from pushing his
Afrika Korps into the Canal Zone with its glittering prizes of
Cairo and Alexandria. On the surface, life went on as usual. The
shops still sold their luxuries, the hotels and nightclubs acted as
though the enemy was only a two-hour motor drive away.

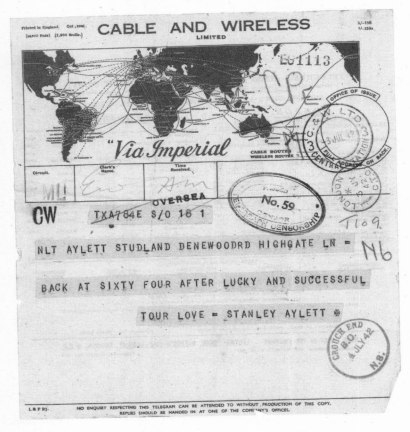

But once again the trains leaving the city were packed. The price of motor cars soared to new levels as anxious European and Egyptian families sought the means to get away, while service wives and various women's services were evacuated to Suez on their way to South Africa. Then, seeing the fleet sail off to less vulnerable points, it was small wonder that the average individual thought the army had little chance of holding the Germans at El Alamein.

At the hospital work and play went on uninterrupted. We knew that whatever happened we were staying on, and with that as a certainty there was no reason why we should interrupt our routine. In subsequent months, if our naval friends became a little expansive over the merits of the navy, we used to remind them playfully that it was the RAMC that had stayed when Alexandria was threatened and that it was the fleet which had steamed away.

The days passed and the line at El Alamein grew stronger. Mussolini, like the dictator of a hundred and forty years ago, had made the mistake of casting medals for a victory that, though it looked certain, was not yet won. The Eighth Army had gained in strength as it fell back on to its great bases whereas the attenuated lines of communication of the enemy, harassed as they were by submarine, warship and aeroplane, proved an increasing embarrassment. Each day that passed was a day lost to Hitler and gained for the Allies.

My small unit was again sent to the desert, to be attached to a CCS sited near the coast behind El Alamein. The few days of inevitable gloom and disappointment we had had when things seemed so critical were rapidly forgotten and once more optimism was in the air. Changes in the army command had brought a completely new atmosphere of confidence. General Montgomery had taken over. There was to be no more retreat. When the enemy attacked he was to be held and then an advance would be prepared. We were to stay where we were and if necessary die where we were. All demoralising uncertainty had gone.

In the months of August and September, changes in the RAMC were taking place, too. The surgical team was enlarged to form the field surgical unit, completely self-contained with regard to operating and surgical equipment and with its own staff car and lorries. True its tentage was not ideal and it had yet to be provided with its own electric-light plant, but it was a step in the right direction, a direction that led to the near perfect unit that finally served with the BLA (British Liberation Army).

For the first time, too, casualty clearing stations in the Middle East were provided with a complement of sisters and they brought increasing efficiency to units that for two years had been without their help. With the exception of those who had served in the hospital at Tobruk, only rarely had British sisters been attached to forward units. But out-of-date ideas and customs were steadily being jettisoned. Although at the beginning nursing regulations at the base still enforced the old traditional uniform, it was not long before it was realised that a sister was still as efficient if she did not wear the scarlet and grey of the Queen Alexandra's Imperial Nursing Service but instead dressed in a far more suitable uniform of khaki slacks and shirt. Somewhere in matronly bosoms at the War Office there must have been much heart-searching, but reason was triumphing over reactionary attitudes.

Until the field surgical unit incorporated the surgical team, we were lucky in having a South African driver who, without the need for any persuasion, had attached himself to us. It was an odd story because for weeks no one in his unit at the base seemed to notice the loss of one of their drivers and his vehicle. He belonged to a South African general-transport company in Alexandria and had been detailed to take my unit up to the desert when we left for the second time. When we had reached our destination and the lorry was unloaded, he proceeded to park it close by and was obviously settling in. On being asked if he was not going to make the journey back that same day, he said, 'I thought I was staying with you. I'm sure my unit will never miss me.'

When we told him this was not our understanding he was terribly upset and asked if he could be allowed to stay. He wanted to serve in the desert and had volunteered to go with any forward unit but still he found himself stationed in Alexandria. This seemed to him an excellent opportunity to achieve his objective. The prospect of having a lorry overcame any conscience we may have had about the matter and we accepted the addition to our strength. With a lorry of our own we were the envy of our less-fortunate fellow units, and moreover our driver turned out to be a first-class reinforcement to our theatre-team strength. We could not have had a more delightful helper.

One day, when our own lorries arrived, we had to say goodbye to him and his now superfluous vehicle. He had been so good that I tried to get him loaned to the RAMC, as there was obviously work there to which he was suited. But I was not successful. I think there were tears in his eyes as he drove away. He had been with us during a busy period when the Germans had put in a desperate last attack to break through the line and had found a job in which he really felt he was pulling his weight. He was very sad at having to leave.

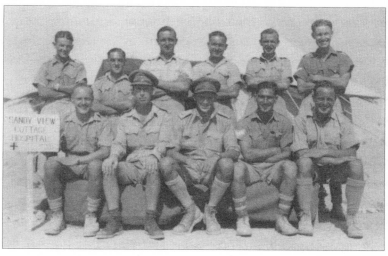

No. 14 Field Surgical Unit (author centre, front row).

Soon after he left us, I too had to go back to the base. I had had dysentery hanging about for some time. You can put up with the odd attack of 'gyppy tummy' but when it gets beyond that stage and your insides feel permanently tied up in knots, the thing becomes different. In the Middle East you get used to visiting the latrine more than the average European, but when you are going at half-hourly intervals and blood gushes out, when you cannot be sure even of arriving in time and when you can hardly stand for weakness, then you should be in hospital. So back I went to my old hospital to lie luxuriously between clean white sheets and to be thoroughly spoiled again while I got better. But I had lost my field surgical unit.

When I was well, after a short period of work at the hospital in which I had been a patient, I once again joined a unit going up to the desert. This CCS was one of two provided with a special surgical unit. It consisted of two enormous lorries, one fitted out as a theatre and the other as a sterilising room. In action these were backed up against one another and linked together by a small gangway. A tarpaulin penthouse supported by a tubular structure running out from the sides of the lorries served the dual purpose of blacking out the junction between the two vehicles and providing additional shelter for patients awaiting surgery. Looking at these ingenious facilities one might well believe that they provided the perfect solution to the needs of a forward surgeon. But in point of fact there were many disadvantages and most of us preferred to operate in a tented theatre. Space, as may be well imagined, was extremely limited and when the surgeon is working in cramped surroundings, the speed of an operation is slowed down. Moreover, time was lost in getting the patient in and out of the lorries and time and speed are both very precious where many wounded are awaiting treatment. In the desert, too, the inside of the vehicles during the hours of darkness, when no windows or ventilators could be opened, became overwhelmingly hot and stuffy. Superficially, they looked magnificent; only when you were working with them did their disadvantages become apparent. Nevertheless, they had been functioning up and down the desert for two years and an enormous amount of fine work had been done in them by previous surgeons and their teams.

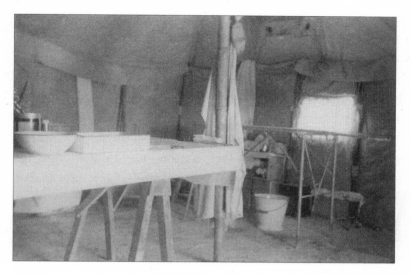

Interior of operating theatre, Sandy View Cottage Hospital, 14 FSU.

One early morning, about a fortnight before the battle of El Alamein, we left our camp at Sidi Bish just on the eastern outskirts of Alexandria. In the bright cool of an early autumn morning the climate in Egypt is perfect. As you drive along the enormous sweeping bay before the glare and blaze of the sun have roused all the flies and dirt and dust, life is as sparkling fresh as the Mediterranean itself.

Travelling towards the desert in the large convoy of a CCS with its forty-odd vehicles stretching far back is somehow thrilling, too. You are sorry to be leaving all the luxuries of a large city, you are sorry in a way to be saying goodbye to hot baths and clean sheets, to good food and pleasant messes. But in spite of all these attractions there are bound to be compensations somewhere out in the desert. There is the possibility of travelling hundreds of miles, of gaining new experience, of seeing new towns and regions. There is more excitement to look forward to away from the routine of the base, where each day is so similar to the one that has gone before.

For a short while you forget that your work is a surgeon's and that ahead lies the prospect of appalling injuries. While the lorry rolls along there is a void and a relaxation from the strain of work and your mind wanders far away into an imagined world. You cannot see all the pain and horror that war brought to so many patients in Alexandria, or the Union Jack-draped bodies that periodically have to be borne out of the wards. Even if you try hard it is difficult to visualise the little room in Tobruk where the dying went. Soon it will all come back, but as you travel along, just for a few hours, you remember all the happy times you had in Alexandria, all the beauty that was in the desert, until it seems that all was happiness and that the tears and disappointments never existed.

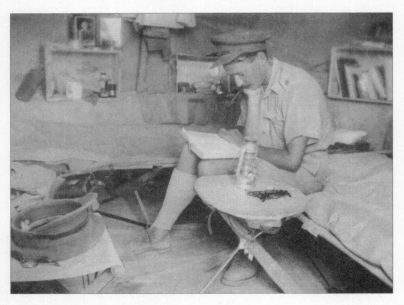

A rare moment alone.

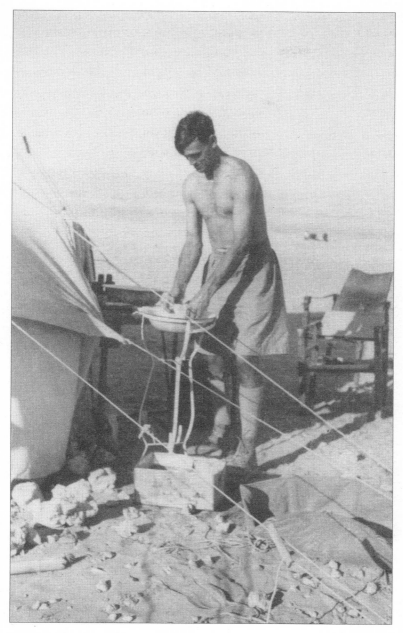

Hygiene routines modified for desert life.

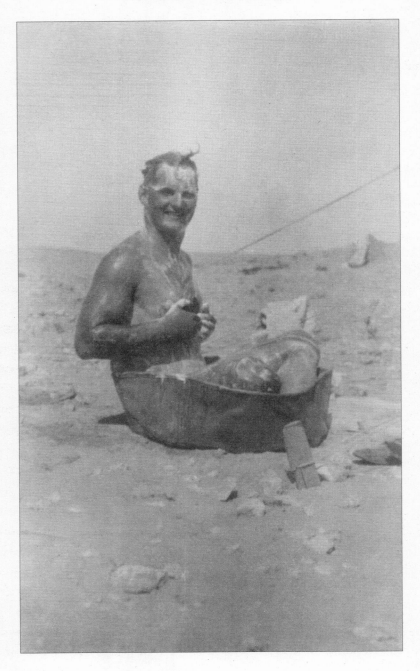

We were going to the southern end of the fifty-mile line that had held the German advance. Here a large concentration of forward medical units was assembled and a small town of tentage had already been set up when we arrived. Perhaps this large medical centre was intended to give further proof to the enemy that the attack was expected to come from the south. I do not know, but when the battle started in the northern sector most of the casualties were evacuated through the casualty clearing stations on the coast, which were filled to overflowing with wounded, whereas the units in the south were comparatively slack.

For about a fortnight before the battle there were of course the few casualties from patrol activities and sporadic shelling and bombing to deal with, but we were busy preparing everything for the day we knew was fast approaching. Then to my intense disappointment, on the day before the battle started I was sent once more back to Alexandria. It was an obvious step to take. By then the RAMC commanders knew it was to the north that their facilities would be strained to capacity, whereas down in the south things would be quiet and easy.

Moreover, with a great base hospital in Alexandria, available within a reasonable distance of the front line, it was obvious that many cases would be sent there for their first surgical treatment. The road back from El Alamein was reasonably good, far better than those leading from the south, and the wounded would not suffer the added ill effects of an extra journey of fifty miles. The urgent cases would be treated by the casualty clearing stations along the evacuation line. All that was needed were additional surgeons and teams to cope with the rush of casualties at the base. So, along with several others, once again I was added to the strength of the hospital.

No. 64 General Hospital was well accustomed to dealing with rushes of casualties. Sisters, orderlies and medical officers knew the routine well. All they needed was to have a few hours' warning and all would be ready. This time, for some unknown reason the warning was not there and the first tide of casualties found the theatres locked, the sterilisers cold. But after a bad start and a lot of adverse comment on the reason for employing senior officers, the hospital was at full stretch. The individual knew full well the part he had to play and even though he grumbled bitterly at the lack of the few hours' warning that could so easily have been given, he soon made up for the delay.

With all the amenities available at a large base hospital, the treatment of the wounded is naturally so much easier than in a forward area. There is no worry about shortages of supplies. Feeding patients from large established kitchens presents none of the problems that arise when a few field-cooking stoves alone are all that are available. Washing facilities and sanitation are already laid on. No problem occurs concerning the water, such as having inadequate quantities for the maintenance of hygiene and sterility, and there is light in all the wards so that you need not grope about in the dim flicker of hurricane lamps. It is still hard work but less exhausting than in a forward surgical centre.

Fifty miles in front of us these latter were working desperately hard in an endeavour to cope with the large number of casualties they were receiving. Periodically, right up to the end of the war, a surgical centre could find itself very short of sisters and surgeons, and under these circumstances – when however hard they worked, the lines of wounded awaiting operation never seemed to diminish – there were few surgeons who did not lose some of their imperturbability. Although in the wards and operating theatres we still managed to maintain evenness and calm, outside we voiced opinions that took no account of crowns or pips, however many of them there might have been.

In our views we were sometimes unfair to those above us. The surgeon only sees a local picture. Of the general overall scheme he is, naturally enough, not told. But when he sees the pre-operative ward filled to overflowing, when he is so tired that it is difficult to keep awake, he wonders why on earth some of his friends, whom he knows are comparatively slack down at the base or in other sectors, are not sent to help him. Or, when visiting the wards, if it is obvious that there are not enough nurses or orderlies even to give all the wounded sufficient drinks, then he has visions of the eighty sisters at each general hospital at the base compared with the few, often exhausted with overwork, attached to the CCS.

Most of our senior officers realised that the suggestions and criticisms that we made were offered in good faith, with only the one idea of somehow improving the lot of the wounded man. One of our finest consulting surgeons used to refer to his forward surgeons as being more temperamental than a bunch of prima donnas. Jokingly he would say that the lot of an operatic producer must be child's play compared with his job of dealing with us, our whims and fancies, our criticisms and demands. But he understood the reason behind them all and knew perhaps that had there been no criticism, no desire to improve, then the surgeon had lost his kindness and his sympathy towards his patients. If that was lost then the incentive to aim at the impossible, which sometimes proved the possible, was also gone.

In Alexandria we welcomed the news of the great British victory at El Alamein with feelings of immense pride and relief. At last the long series of reverses and retreats was being forgotten in an overwhelming enemy defeat. Even the German naval officer, who a few weeks before had said to the sister looking after him, 'Field Marshal Rommel will be here in a few days, but do not be frightened, he is a perfect gentleman', was looking glum and dispirited, while the newer wounded prisoners had lost some of the arrogance of those who had been with us before.

As the weeks went by, those who had fled from Alexandria came trickling back. Politely, we made no reference to their absence and no enquiries as to what South Africa was like. The city, with the threat of occupation by the enemy averted, was rapidly returning to its normal carefree ways. Only those few who had foreseen the prospect of much loot and plunder in the days or hours during the changeover from one army to another were disappointed. However, there were still enormous numbers of British troops left, anxious to be parted from their money.

Nov. 8 No. 64 General Hospital, MEF

My dear Mum and Dad

What grand news. At last it has come after all these months of waiting and hoping, and after all our very bitter disappointments. What an indescribable feeling of relief that at last the army has justified itself – has scored a victory to put it side by side with the navy and the RAF. It is absolutely grand. And I only wish I had been in the 8th Army's victory as well as in the defeat previously. No matter. The beginning of the end appears in sight...

The Axis armies are in full retreat. I know well what retreat means. But when to it is added air superiority it must be terrible. When we came back fortunately we had air superiority... but now hell must be let loose on those roads – awful terrifying hell with no escape from incessant, everlasting attack. One cannot but be glad. They deserve it. And yet one cannot but imagine well the sight of mangled bodies, wrenched limbs and torn flesh and in friend or foe. I'm tired of that sight.

Love, Stanley

Dec. 17 No. 64 Gen. Hosp.

Dear Mum and Dad

I know that I have had my share of luck and perhaps a bit of someone else's as well. And I hope we may all fare as well in the future.

I was very pleased to hear from my ex-patient, Turner. He was really a grand lad as all New Zealanders are, and I do not think I have ever seen such an ill man recover. He had what is called gas gangrene and for days hovered with more than one leg in the grave. In fact we thought he'd got both in on more than one occasion, but what with his struggles and mine and other peoples he managed to climb out again.

No I don't regard it as a feather in my cap. Just an enormous sense of relief fills me when now and then a battle that appears hopeless is won. Hard bruised that I am, I am afraid that on occasions I have almost wept over the appallingness of shattered men. I know that I am good at this war surgery. That is not conceit – it is just a fact and if I can get a chap well, that is satisfaction enough for me. I'm not in the slightest bit interested in success for success's sake.

Love, Stanley

Christmas and a happy – a very happy – New Year came. True, in the autumn, the bad weather had saved the Afrika Korps from encirclement and complete destruction, true the Eighth Army was being held up by lines of defence back upon which the enemy was falling, but in spite of these minor matters there was an atmosphere of supreme confidence in final victory among all those returning from the desert with whom we came in contact. Our rush of casualties had ceased. Once again the hospital was reverting to its true base functions and for a while I was sent back to the desert.

In the winter the desert was not always filled with sunshine. Often heavy rain poured down so that the hospital tents lay in a bed of sandy mud. It was bitterly cold too, and no greatcoats or mufflers were adequate protection against biting winds. Canvas wards were difficult to heat sufficiently with the few oil stoves we had at our disposal, but in bed, wrapped up in many blankets, the patients could be kept reasonably comfortable.

One night a wandering Senussi woman came in with her husband. She was already well into her labour but some difficulties had arisen and so reluctantly she had come to us. We had no other place to put her but in one of our ordinary wards filled with lightly wounded, behind some screens to separate her bed from the rest of our patients. Soon the child's cries announced to a thrilled ward full of soldiers that in the midst of suffering and death there was still new life. There was almost disappointment when, within a few hours of her delivery, the mother, with her newborn child, insisted on leaving us. We could not explain any of the dangers. We did not speak her language, and no doubt even if we could have done, the result would have been the same. So from the very first day she introduced her infant to a hard life on the borderline of starvation in which only the fittest survive.

To these natives, somehow extracting an existence from the poor desert soil, war brought a catalogue of dangers. Sometimes they became involved in desert battles or bombing attacks, at others they would, unknowingly, wander out on to minefields or among booby traps. Their children, finding some attractive piece of metal, would pick it up to take it as a toy. Sometimes these bright toys would be detonators or grenades. There would be a flash and only the stumps of bones would push out to show where a moment before a leg or hand had been.

Most of the desert casualty clearing stations would have several such patients. Sometimes we evacuated them down to the civilian hospitals in Alexandria, but this was never a popular move with the relatives, however severely injured the child may have been, and now and then they insisted on taking them away. Occasionally we would see the child again with its wounds encased in the mud-and-dung dressing of primitive medical practice.

Spring comes early in Egypt and for a few brief weeks the edge of the desert is coloured with flowers of every hue, pushing their way through sand and gravel. The unit I was working with now had no need for an extra surgeon and again I was sent back to my hospital in Alexandria. Here the winter rains had washed away all the dust and dirt and the gardens and parks were vivid with startling colour.

In that year of 1943, as the races and creeds across the Middle East were celebrating this feast of spring and welcoming the return of life, a series of victories hundreds of miles away in Tripolitania foreshadowed the end of the war which for three years now had ebbed and flowed along the desert miles. Now there was only the aftermath of battle in the hospitals far away at the base, and life turned back three years to almost pre-war conditions.

For us, there was the routine of work of the civilian type, though occasionally some minor naval action would bring in casualties. But now, with many large hospitals far up towards the forward areas, the days of treating urgent battle casualties were over.

14

WORK IN A PLASTIC UNIT AND NO. 10 CCS

JUNE–DECEMBER 1943

From Alexandria to a plastic-surgery unit in Cairo; No. 10 Casualty Clearing Station outside Tobruk; unexpected return to Glasgow

For a little while, this easy life could not have been more pleasant. We worked in the mornings and in the early hours of the evenings, and in those periods had more than enough time to do our job. The afternoons could be filled with sailing or tennis, golf or bathing, and in the later hours of the day, when even the blackout regulations had been relaxed, were all the pleasures in Alexandria which had largely disappeared from the big cities in Europe.

Holidays from hard work could be too long, however. The urge to be in the forward areas, where, in some small part at least, one could share the life of the fighting troops and care for their battle casualties, returned. The easy life could not be lived with any contentment when the more difficult beckoned. Few young and fit men serving in the armed forces enjoyed for more than a short while the life of comparative comfort, and of those who, because of their particular work, had to stay at the base nearly all envied their comrades in the forward areas. The latter, who referred disparagingly and vulgarly to the 'fucking base wallahs with their velvet-arsed jobs', had no real ambition to exchange their own.

When finally, months later, we left for England a regiment was going home whose men had seen little fighting service. It was no fault of their own. They had lost their tanks in a ship on its way to the Middle East and for a very long time replacements failed to materialise. Instead of being delighted with the good fortune which had kept them out of battle and which had eliminated their chance of becoming casualties they were, on the contrary, very disgruntled with the way chance had treated them.

But for the ravages of a minute bacillus, *Shigella dysenteriae*, which had reduced me and all my intestines to a temporary wreck, the easy life would not have been mine. I should have been travelling through Benghazi and Tripoli with my field surgical unit and up into the mainland of Italy. For three and a half years I had worked with battle casualties. That was my life and my speciality. It was a type of surgery very different from that of civilian practice. It was surgery in the raw, the immediate repair of damage, self-inflicted by a warring world, and very different from that required for the cure of natural disease. It was carried out in makeshift surroundings and not in the ordered calm of shiningly clean operating theatres of a peacetime environment. It required, too, immediate decisions without any preliminary investigations or ancillary aids to diagnosis.

I wondered about the future. My original endeavours and ambitions had been directed towards becoming a consultant surgeon, perhaps in my own teaching hospital. This required prolonged academic study as well as a rigorous ongoing training given to me by my masters and chiefs. It required also the passing of still higher and more advanced degrees, those only those of my contemporaries still in England were able to sit and acquire. I saw an uncertain future after the war, if I survived to its end – and I had had my brushes with death – but that end was far away. For the present I knew that in forward-battle surgery I was at my best and could offer most, but the armies had achieved their end in the Middle East and North Africa and the war had entered the continent of Europe. I was hundreds of miles away.

About this time a circular came round asking for volunteers from the RAMC to join the Parachute Regiment and I applied, only to be told that recruitment was open only to general-duty officers and not to surgical specialists. I approached Sir Heneage Ogilvie, then consultant surgeon to the Middle East forces, who understood and appreciated very well my feelings, but in his command there were no forward units and postings to other theatres of war had to come from England. However, as the work at No. 64 General Hospital had become so light and was likely to remain so, and as I was supernumerary to the unit's establishment, he suggested I be posted to Cairo to be attached to the plastic-surgery unit there, and from thence sent to a CCS working as a line-of-communication unit in the desert.

I left No. 64 General Hospital for the final time. I had formed a deep respect and affection for this unique army and the navy hospital that had so often been involved in the initial treatment of casualties from all the services. There, no inter-service rivalry had ever existed, and from the commanding officer downwards the one aim of all had been how best to look after and rehabilitate our wounded and sick patients. There too, I had my first experiences in the surgery of tropical diseases, typhoid fever, which silently eroded the bowel to perforation and which responded dramatically to none of the drugs then available, and *amoebiasis*, which again infected the intestine and spread to ulcerate the liver, so producing abscesses that required drainage.

Alexandria, too, had cast its spell. Its wonderful beaches, its colour and life in spite of the poverty, its mixture of nations from Europe and the Levant and other parts of Africa, its history stretching back to a great civilisation that had housed the finest library in the world, its position at the junction of east and west where the twain did meet, all made it a city one could not leave without some regret.

I arrived in Cairo and found a bed in the National Hotel. It was never a question of finding a *room* in this crowded capital, where even a single unit had to accommodate at least three, just a *space*. The following morning I searched around for something more permanent, and in the outer part of Cairo at Heliopolis found a small service flat. Years had passed since I had had a room to myself and been on my own, and on this first evening I wallowed in the luxury, not even troubling to go out. I had for a time an awful feeling that I would like this life too much and become a proper base wallah.

Next morning I reported to the unit to which I was to be attached. It was in a hospital the like of which I had not seen for years. The wards were fly-proofed, there was no dust or sand and the operating theatres were insulated against the heat. There was no rush and no shortage of staff; sterile operating gowns were in abundance and there was none of the make-do-and-mend of the forward surgeon. The unit was under the direction of Major Michael Oldfield, who before the war had been a consultant in plastic surgery at Leeds. Now he was restoring shattered faces with pieces of bone removed from the soldier's pelvis, refashioning noses and ears with fragments of cartilage, covering destroyed tissue with grafts stepped up in stages towards the final area where they were to provide the new skin covering, gently removing the contracted tissues of limbs which had been incinerated, and suturing over these raw areas sheets of skin taken from some other part of the body to restore the joint's mobility. He was a superb technical surgeon and his work, so time-consuming and meticulous, never faltered. His unit was a miniature of the famed and magnificent one at East Grinstead in England, but it was a superb miniature. For over a month I had the benefit of his teaching, which was to stand me in such good stead in the future and for which I was to remain always grateful.

The evening time was free. We sipped drinks on the veranda at Shepheard's, went to open-air cinemas and danced at the Mena Palace Hotel, with the Sphinx and the Pyramids close by silhouetted against the deep dark blue of the desert sky. I said farewell to a precious friend with a heart that ached as only that of a lover can. Years had gone by since I had sent her red roses for remembrance when she, a nurse, had sailed from England. I had written letters which had not arrived and my last, of such desperate importance to us both, directed and redirected and delayed for many months, arrived on her return from her honeymoon. I never saw her again, but at least on that last night I had persuaded her to rejoin the Army Nursing Service where her compassion and skill, her beauty and her tenderness must have brought encouragement and hope to the wounded for whom she cared in the Italian campaign.

I did receive one letter – at least an envelope that contained simply a poem by Alice Meynell.

I must not think of thee: and, tired yet strong,
I shun the thought that lurks in all delight –
The thought of thee – and in the blue heaven's height,
And in the sweetest passage of a song.

Oh, just beyond the fairest thoughts that throng
This breast, the thought of thee waits hidden yet bright:
But it must never, never come in sight;
I must stop short of thee the whole day long.

But when sleep comes to close each difficult day,
When night gives pause to the long watch I keep,
And all my bonds I needs must loose apart,
Must doff my will as raiment laid away –
With the first dream that comes with the first sleep
I run, I run, I am gathered to thy heart.

After about four weeks I received a posting order to join No. 10 casualty clearing station, a unit in which briefly I had served in 1940. The train from Cairo slowly puffed its way north through the delta and then joined the newly constructed line that led miles into the desert. At the railhead I stayed in a transit camp for the night and the following day a truck took me to my new unit. I was glad that once more I was away from the base.

The tents of the CCS came into view stretched out on the cliffs above a cobalt sea some ten miles outside Tobruk. For some weeks it had been without a lieutenant-colonel, and from the major who was acting in command I took over until the new CO arrived from England. It seemed strange that the RAMC division of the War Office should think it necessary to send someone out from England when there were so many first-class men in the casualty clearing stations and field ambulances who had spent years learning the art of desert life and navigation. To the simple mind of a civilian in uniform it appeared reasonable to suppose a person like that was far more likely to prove a successful CO of a desert unit than someone who for the last three years had been at home in England. But the reasonable way was not to be and we waited expectantly for our new arrival. We knew that whoever he was he would have much to live up to; the previous CO, an old rugby international, had become almost a legend in the unit.

Our work was mainly concerned with looking after the local sick of the comparatively large Tobruk garrison, although from a surgical point of view there were always the accidental injuries, usually resulting from hidden landmines or grenades. To the end we never really understood the function of the large number of troops there and we always wondered whether anyone else did either.

One of its more important jobs seemed to be concerned with building a hospital, the purpose of which was completely lost on us. Because of its site we knew that it was surely going to be flooded when the rains came and that it would certainly be a white elephant. We had seen others, badly placed, going up before. In any case the war was across the seas now. The wounded were not going to be ferried across the Mediterranean to this desolate spot, and among local troops a small unit was well able to deal with their injuries and illnesses. However, we looked after the health of the prisoners of war and engineers who were building it and the RASC companies supplying the transport. To feed us in our great work a contingent of bakers baked bread for us all.

Somehow No. 10 CCS had been left behind in the general advance, and instead of serving in its proper place dealing with battle casualties it had been stranded on lines of communication which, now the war had left North Africa, seemed scarcely necessary. However, in no small measure due to our nurses, it was a happy and efficient unit, and with an eye to a future in more active conditions, free hours were often spent pitching and re-pitching tents and setting out various types of operating theatres in am endeavour to make ourselves still more proficient.

One day an ambulance drew up to the unit and a rather elderly and fragile officer alighted. He looked so unwell that we were just going to take him along to the wards when he announced that he was our new CO. We were thunderstruck. However quiet conditions are in the desert from a battle point of view, living still demands a reasonable physique and good health and our new CO we felt had neither. Nevertheless, we welcomed him warmly.

The unit quickly named him 'the Sheriff'. Somehow he looked just like a sheriff who had stepped out of a Hollywood Western, especially as he wore his belt so loosely that it fell down over his hips as if supporting the heavy weight of two loaded revolvers. He was a Scot, in fact the only Scot of the comic stereotype that I have ever met. He wasn't going to waste money buying officer-style shirts and went about in those designed for other ranks, and he had a flair for collecting small pieces of soap wherever he saw them and making them into a large cake. In spite of his oddities and the fact that we knew he would not last long, we liked him. But it seemed a pity that we had to alter the routine of the unit, which was good, because it did not conform to exercises theoretically performed somewhere in the region of Salisbury Plain.

He was by no means without a sense of humour, and that is the most valuable of all assets in a unit which for weeks and months on end has little outside entertainment and so becomes dependent on its personalities. On one of his rare visits a local senior colonel of the RAMC, whom we considered somewhat pompous and ineffective, was having tea in the mess. In his broadest Scots accent our colonel said, 'Ah see you're wearin' the territorial decoration like myself. In my home town they call it the badge of shame and say it comes just before a bowler hat.' We laughed appreciatively, looking meaningfully at the visiting colonel. He, however, saw nothing funny in this disrespect of his medal or the suggestion of what was likely to follow, and maintained a stony stare.

Not long after his arrival, a really hot spell descended upon us and the colonel took it badly. He looked exhausted and we all felt rather sorry for him. There were surely plenty of younger and fitter men at home who could have come before this man wearing the honourable ribbons of the last war. It really seemed amazing that the choice should have fallen on him. Not long after, he became really ill and was invalided home. I think he was glad to go because he knew he was not fit enough for the job, but as he left he told us how sorry he was to be leaving such a first-class unit.

While awaiting another CO we continued our training programme, exercising with compass and map in the surrounding desert. Games and competitions were organised with other units and with this added impetus we did not grow stale and dull. On a line-of-communication job it is very easy to fall into a routine that, because of its daily sameness and monotony, induces slackness and inefficiency. This fortunately we avoided. Now and then we had the excitement of an ENSA show and periodically the Army Film Unit would visit. So the days and weeks passed by until we began to wonder whether we were ever going to have a colonel or be transferred away from this quiet life.

It was not surprising that some of the best and most active of our nursing orderlies should have asked for a transfer to a unit engaged in any theatre in the world as long as it was in the forward areas. To me this seemed a reasonable enough request. I had felt the same down at the base and would have welcomed a change to a harder life. It was not that these men were not happy in this casualty clearing station, but they felt that somewhere else they could be of more use, and of course they were right.

So the applications were duly forwarded to the colonel with the 'badge of shame' and the lack of humour. I was amazed at his reply, but I suppose an absent sense of humour usually betokens an absence of human understanding as well. There was a point blank refusal to consider the applications, which in his opinion showed that the discipline and morale of the unit were bad and should at once be tightened up.

As I read the letter, I became very angry. All of us I think were very proud of the unit. We knew it was good, and capable of a far better job than it was now being called upon to perform. For someone who paid it only the rarest of visits and really had no idea of its merits or vices, to judge a unit in this way was unjust in the extreme. Red tabs and pips and crown or not, his criticism was not going unanswered. I pointed out in my reply that his allegations had not the slightest basis in truth, and because a man volunteered for a forward job there was no reason for morale and discipline to come under suspicion. I added that when I had tried to get into the Paratroops, I had not considered that either my morale or the discipline of the hospital to which I was attached were open to question. Perhaps it was rather a heated letter from an officer of considerably junior rank, but there are certain occasions when discretion has to be abandoned if the cause is just. However, I heard no more of the matter. Subsequently the CCS came to prove itself one of the finest in the British Army.

At last our new colonel arrived, bringing with him the news of an impending move. No news could have been more exciting. We had no idea where we were going – to Italy, Burma, India… ? We could have speculated for hours on all the possibilities. The unit was enthusiastic over the prospects to a man. The colonel soon went down to Cairo where he was to receive further orders. As he was not returning but was joining us in the Canal Zone, I again took over command.

Some days after he left, a rumour spread throughout the unit like a sudden sandstorm, blowing up from who knew where. We were going home to England. Where the rumour originated was impossible to trace, but it was a rumour that, however improbable, somehow appeared to have the hallmark of veracity. Then, like pieces of a jigsaw puzzle, small happenings and events all seemed to fit into the picture of the story of a move back home. Officers who had not been long in the country were exchanged for old-timers. Winter kit was issued to the men and all our medical stores and

Subject:- Transfers - Other Ranks.

To:- A.D.M.S.,
    99th., Sub-Area,
    Middle East Forces.

No. 10 (Mob) C. C. S.,
M. E. F.
Reference, 10CCS/3/35.b.

2nd., November, 1943.

Reference H.Q. Cyrenaica District letter, CYR/3/M., dated
29th., Oct., 43., forwarded under cover of your letter, ref:
100S/M., dated 1st., November, 1943.

1.   I have noted the remarks in your letter.

2.   This Unit has served for nearly 12 months in an L of C
capacity, and it's discipline and morale, in spite of this, is
of the highest standard and will compare with any R.A.M.C.,
formation. I do not think that it needs any investigation.

3.   It is the first time that I have known a reflection to
be directed towards a Unit because some of it's members wish
to share the more adverse conditions of a forward Company in
whichever part of the globe to which they may be sent.
When I applied from a Base Hospital to join a Field Surgical
Unit and then the Paratroops, I did not feel that it was a
reflection on my personal discipline or morale. I feel the
same about these men, who are very excellent.

4.   This unfounded slight is most unfair and unjust and is
a reflection not only on the men, but particularly on the
Officers most of whom have recently been posted away.

S.O. Aylett

(S.O. Aylett) Major, R.A.M.C.,
for, Officer Commanding 10th (Mob) C.C.S.

Field.
jo/-

The author's reply of 2 November 1943 to the ADMS 99th Sub-Area, MEF.

tentage were to be handed in. The latter took days to check with
the local quartermaster, who remained convinced we should have
had a lot more. We could hardly be going to Italy if we were to
leave our equipment behind. What did not fit into the picture was
the fact that we were issued with mosquito nets and anti-malarial
Mepacrine tablets. We finally came to the conclusion after a long
discussion that this must be a red herring.

219

Oct. 20 No. 10 Mobile CCS

Dear Mum and Dad,

Outside the wind is roaring. Brilliant lightning is flashing in the sky making the night like day. The whole camp is a quagmire the result of two days heavy rain, and the thunder is rumbling away. And yet my spirit and that of the unit runs high. What does the rain and the wind matter. To hell with the lightning and the storm. At last we've to do a job of work. That is the only thing that matters and although perhaps not just at the minute the prospect is there. The past, with the hum drum monotony of sand and scrub is passed. Almost forgotten, soon a myth and only the happy moments will stand out and colour its memory. Well and happy it is that the bad moments are so easily lost in the sea of one's memory because there have been moments when one has wondered how life could be endured with its futility and waste of time, its discomfort and boredom.

Once again I am CO (temporarily) of the unit. At such a time there is a lot to do arranging this, sorting out the problems that arrive all through the day at such a time of flux as this. But I quite like organising work and I do not find it boring as some people seem to do. There are many times when I think that from the team point of view I should have been a chartered accountant or a lawyer instead of a surgeon, as a lot of my time is with accounts and attending to legislative details. You cannot appreciate the amount of correspondence that a unit such as this deals with and I must sign my name a hundred times a day.

The day for the move was appointed and a fleet of three-tonners arrived to move us down to a camp near Alexandria. It was a journey of three days by lorry. With an early start, a staff car could do it in a day or at the most a day and a half. It was strange, therefore, that no staff cars were made available for our sisters; instead they were obliged to travel by lorry. That there were a considerable number of cars in Alexandria, not engaged in what could be called essential duties, was undoubted, but to the last, save in certain corps and administrations, it rarely seemed to be the policy of the RAMC to look after its nursing staff to the fullest degree possible. Even after the war in Europe was over, many were sent back to England from the Continent in various types of landing craft, which, to say the least, were ill-equipped for the transport of women on a trip lasting many hours. This attitude seemed peculiar to the British Army for it was not found in the Dominion forces. Undoubtedly no sister wished to be pampered – they would have resented this treatment had it been offered to them – but there were many simple arrangements that could have made all the difference to their comfort.

This journey down from Tobruk was a typical example. Along the desert miles, flat and featureless, there are none of the friendly copses and dells of a European countryside. Even in wartime, when sensibilities are reduced, it was more than a little embarrassing for the sisters to know that at the various halts a little squad of men had to be assembled with spades, buckets and hessian to erect a ladies' restroom close to a long cavalcade of lorries. Life at times for the forward nurses was raw, but when it was necessary they did not mind and welcomed the opportunity to cope as best they could. It was only when it was obviously uncalled for and could have been avoided with some thought and consideration that it became hurtful.

Outside Alexandria we were accommodated in a section of a vast camp. The town was out of bounds except for those on duty, but fortunately, for a medical officer there are always very good reasons that take him to the local hospital and thus enable him to escape any restrictions. You want to X-ray a man's chest, to arrange for some massage or other physiotherapy, or else to take him in for consultation with another specialist at the base hospital, and naturally enough the patient is delighted to make the trip. From a security point of view it would have made no difference. There were vast numbers of Egyptians wandering around the camp, and a crowd of transports assembled in the harbour were there for all to see. Where we were going we did not know, our guess was as good as anyone else's, but that a move was in progress was obvious. Just in case it was to be England, we bought dozens and dozens of oranges and lemons on any trips into town.

Soon, not even on duty were we allowed to leave, and a day came when we were told that we would be embarking on the following morning. Our money was changed and we knew for certain we were bound for England when we saw the pile upon pile of new English banknotes to be exchanged for our tattered piastres. Mosquito nets and Mepacrine tablets were handed in. Our return home, which not a few weeks ago had looked to be years away, had come suddenly and unexpectedly.

As slowly we drew away from the harbour and the buildings on the waterfront became a hazy outline in the distance, all the excitement of going home suddenly fell away. It was to return soon, but for the present the poignant memories of three long years came to the fore. It was three years of youth that we were leaving behind in Egypt and the desert, and to some these years had held all the sadness and sweet happiness of their short lifetimes. We were leaving friends behind as well, lying beneath the little crosses that are scattered through the desert in clusters like small oases.

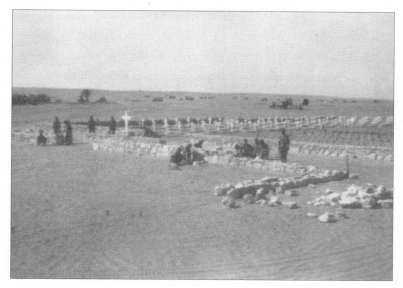

Desert cemetery.

Memory is kind in its forgetfulness. The filth and dirt and sadness of war and the tears that, however hard you tried, welled up into your eyes uncontrollably, faded into the distance as rapidly as the shoreline on the horizon. Already it was becoming an effort to recollect those times when the dawn of each day was welcome only because it brought relief from the lines of ambulances pouring in during the hours of darkness. Already that little room in Tobruk where the dying went was losing its tragedy and its inexpressible loneliness. Instead it was the times of happiness that stood out, coloured and very near. For some there were memories of the perfect and exquisite love that above all else these years of war had brought.

It was a happy ship, and one that was homeward bound. Although we had no illusions as to why we were being sent home, although we knew full well that ahead lay an Allied operation of unprecedented proportions, for the present it was enough to think that by Christmastime we should be reunited with our families. The future that lay beyond that could look after itself.

In the convoy there were many ships that had sailed out with us. They weren't the spic-and-span ships we had seen three years before; constant voyaging with little opportunity or time for refitting had seen to that. But the familiar outlines were there just the same. We recognised the *Samaria* and the *Franconia*, the *Monarch of Bermuda* and the portly contours of the *Drunken Duchess*, for whom we all had a vague feeling of regard. Her behaviour was always erratic and spectacular and it came as no surprise to any of us to see her inflict a glancing blow on her boyfriend the *Monarch*. She sailed proudly onward, but the *Monarch* had to put back to port to repair the damage he had suffered from the wayward *Duchess*. Soon she was to be elevated in the aristocracy of ships to the rank of *Empress*, and perhaps would forsake the carefree ways of the lower peerage.

★ ★ ★

One early morning before the light of a December morning had stolen over the hills, we came slowly into the Clyde. It seemed bitterly cold but we did not mind – we were home. Already the dawn was lighting up green hills and fields, and from scattered homes lights were twinkling as the hours of blackout ended. Slowly, very slowly, the scene of which we had dreamed was taking shape and colour. We watched like excited schoolboys at their first theatre. It was so green, so quiet, so unruffled, as if it knew nothing of war. Three years ago we had said goodbye and now we had come back. The scene was blessedly familiar; it had not changed and we had not forgotten it, not one fragment.

We were moored at last. The customs came aboard. 'I'm afraid you will have to parade your men. We don't like it with you chaps home after years abroad, but we have to do it,' said the officer. 'I want you to ask them in front of me whether any of them has more than five hundred cigarettes.' He gave me a look that is of the type that is as good as a nod. He knew as well as I knew that most of us had about two thousand each. I paraded the men. 'There is no one among you, is there, who has more than five hundred cigarettes?' said I pointedly to my unit. The lines stood firm. A look of complete innocence on all but one face. He was having a big battle with his conscience or else had not taken my question in the way in which it was intended. After a pause he stepped forward. The customs officer hastily found a friend to whom he had something urgent to say. I looked the other way until a sharp yelp of pain announced that a well-placed kick from one of his comrades had brought him to his senses. When I looked back again the line was once again straight and regular. 'No officer,' I said. 'There is no one with more than five hundred cigarettes.'

We were allowed off the ship now. On the quay everyone sought out the telephone boxes and queues soon formed, each man waiting his turn to ring home. In a few seconds you would be talking to your family. Just now they were probably having breakfast, little guessing that you were waiting to telephone them here — here, home in Britain. Perhaps they were wondering when they were going to hear from you again, because weeks ago you had written to tell them not to worry if the mail did not reach them for some time. Naturally enough they would have assumed you were being sent out to India or Burma. That you were coming home could never have crossed their minds.

As the queue waited, there was the self-conscious talk over trivialities that the Englishman always uses to hide the excitement of emotion that he so rarely allows any degree of normal expression. You knew that in spite of all the apparent calmness each man's heart was beating a little faster as he wondered what it was going to be like to talk to his wife or sweetheart, his father or mother, after those years that had changed so much. You knew that the man in front and the man behind had just the same feeling as you somewhere inside his stomach. He was smoking hard, like yourself, but that was the only sign he gave of the excitement that was twisting his very bowels.

At last your turn came. In your ear you heard the burr–burr of the telephone bell ringing hundreds of miles away. They must have been wondering who was ringing them up so early in the morning. Then there was the voice at the other end.

'Hello,' I said. 'This is Stanley speaking. I've come home.'

15

CHRISTMAS AT HOME AND PREPARATIONS FOR D-DAY

DECEMBER 1943–JUNE 1944

Family reunion in London; ordered to Cambridge to prepare
No. 10 Casualty Clearing Station for D-Day; appointed
to command No. 14 Field Surgical Unit

W e went to a reception office, gave the address of where we would be staying, received a travel warrant and some food coupons and were sent on leave for three weeks. Instructions as to where we were to rejoin our unit would be posted to us. Most of us, at least initially, were going to London, and we boarded the train. Almost three years ago, a lifetime ago it seemed, I had piled out of a similar carriage with different companions to join the *Nea Hellas*, sailing in convoy for Suez.

Christmas 1943, and rations were at their most meagre, yet somehow my mother managed to make dinner a feast. Down in the cellar were saved a few bottles of champagne and of whisky, too, for such an occasion and these father brought out. Oranges

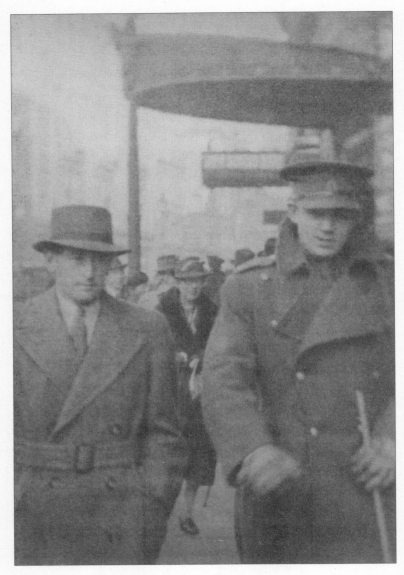

On leave in London, before the invasion of Normandy.

and lemons from the Middle East were heaped in a bowl in the centre of the table. My deep suntan contrasted with the pallor of my parents and of those of my relatives who had come to this reunion. Life had been very difficult for all of them. The loosening threads of the family affairs were knitted back together. My parents' happiness would have been complete had it not been that very much in their thoughts was my brother, recovering from severe wounds received when his ship had been torpedoed. After dinner my car was taken off its blocks and it started with little reluctance. A temporary licence would have to be obtained but with the petrol coupons that were a leave allocation I would be mobile.

In reunions with families and friends and the return to old haunts, the future was forgotten in three weeks of carefree leave. Now and then you would dimly realise that the days were flying by, but it was an unpleasant thought and one that was quickly banished. For a few weeks you escaped from all reality into a blinkered present that put away thoughts of the death and destruction you had seen and that you knew was still proceeding unhindered in so many parts of the globe.

Three weeks was too short a time to bridge the gap of years, save with your dearest friends. Somewhere inside was a gash that war had made, as real as the vicious wound that laid open a man's entrails, though there was not a mark on the skin. You had imagined that as soon as you were home all the inner turmoil would disappear, but soon you realised that there was no shortcut to a cure. Only when sanity returned to an insane world would that gash heal. Healing would come with peace, but peace lay beyond the long months ahead. For the present you could only bandage the gash mentally by forgetting it as best as you could.

During this time I wrote two letters to my great friend and fellow doctor, John Gilpin.

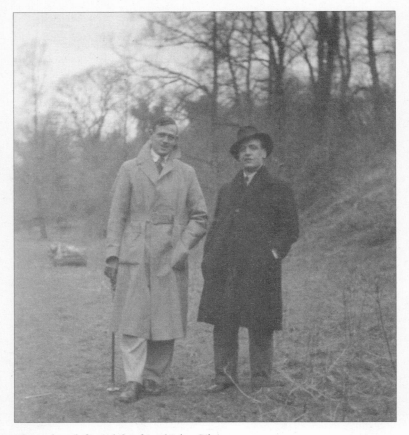

The author (left) with his friend John Gilpin.

26 Jan. 10 CCS, 2 Cranmer Road, Cambridge

My dear John,

I felt that I might just as well have been dropping in for one of our periodic meetings rather than seeing you for the first time for over 3½ years. It was I say again a grand two nights and a day and you could not have picked a more sweet and charming companion for me. Yes you are right. Sweetness and loveliness and genuineness seem rather to have disappeared during this war and it is definitely rare to find it. Let us hope that for both of us the search and the achievement will come soon to us, because without it we can never be truly and really happy.

Guy I saw and loved his company again. But almost embittered he is against existing things. In this I can sympathise so well and had I been all the time in England I should have felt the same. As it is I am a very vivid shade of red. I feel so strongly that at the end of this war unless we fight tooth and nail, once more shall we be taken for a ride that will lead to another Munich in 1969. I do not believe much in the sincerity of most of our leaders or of the big powers behind the scenes. I think that all they wish for is a retention of the old ways, even by the expense of blood in this present conflict.

When I see the Banks paying dividends of 14% and showing a profit of 1½ million pounds on the year's work, and on the other side, in my own corps, a charitable fund for the aid of widows and orphans of the troops who have been killed, in the war I wonder what it is all about. When I read in a shipping company's report that they have had the best year for many years, and hope to do equally well in the following year, when dead bodies wash ashore at Alexandria eaten away by fishes, whilst ships sink – sink with men alive like you and I aboard – then I feel like vomiting. When I know that there is a spirit of idealism abroad, amongst so many, idealism that spells freedom and fairness and when I know the forces, the powers for selfishness and control that it will have to fight, I often wonder. For myself I am convinced that only by nationalisation of all capital can we build a happy England.

24 March 14 Field Surgical Unit, 21 Cranmer Rd, Cambridge

Dear John,

I cannot see amongst my colleagues in this and in any of the other units that, married or single, they have any contentment or peace. For a few brief days when you're on leave you try to pretend that you're far away from it all, back to normality, back to most of what one hoped for and wished for. But always there is the shadow in the future. There is no escape from it, no really going so far away that it cannot work the brief happiness one lives in. Not till all is over and finished can we live and return to a contented spirit and a happy mind because whilst this war is on the search for that is I think quite hopeless. Perhaps you and I may think we could find it, if we were married, anchored to something more than to what we are. But I still think that we should be sadly disillusioned, and good thing though it would be, we should have that sense of non-achievement and frustration still with us.

Soon and surely soon all this war will have ended and then, happy day, we can start to truly live and not exist.

We went to Cambridge to rejoin our casualty clearing station and mobilise in the early weeks of January. I think we were glad to see each other once again because this little world of ours, so small, so temporary, was now the one in which we fitted best. Outside we were for the most part visitors, holidaying among strangers. Here we knew each other so well. Vices and virtues, failures and triumphs had no need to be hidden away. Indeed, during the months we had lived together, sometimes those matters nearest to our hearts were eased by conversation. We recognised the troubles and sympathised, understood the successes and were thrilled and pleased.

It was good to see our Irish friends again, for a time more at home with us than in their neutral country across the sea. One was a giant of a man, almost as large in girth as a famous Irish newspaper peer and not unlike him in other ways. He had been blown up at El Alamein, but a shattered foot now perpetually swollen with oedema was not going to prevent him from going across to France if he could possibly help it. To his dismay he had been considered unfit for service during the early days of the invasion and was transferred from our unit, but somehow – how we never really understood – he arrived on the beaches at Arromanches with one of the first RAMC units to land. He was immensely delighted to be there before us.

Back from Ireland also came his friend Captain Lynham. Without the delightful uncertainties of his Gaelic temperament the unit would not have been the same. He was our mess secretary and his fear of eternal damnation could not have been worse than the terrible anxiety that overcame him on the approach of audit day. 'If mess members will not sign their chits, oi'll not carry on,' Paddy would complain indignantly at the end of one of his sessions with the figures. 'Sorry, Paddy,' we would say to this wizard who had achieved a balance. 'We'll be most careful in the future', and for a time we were, until in the heat of a midnight argument once again the bar chits went unsigned. Then, from scraps of paper, scribbled entries and improvised receipts that should have been there but were not, a maze of figures that somehow added up emerged from a pile of cigarette ends.

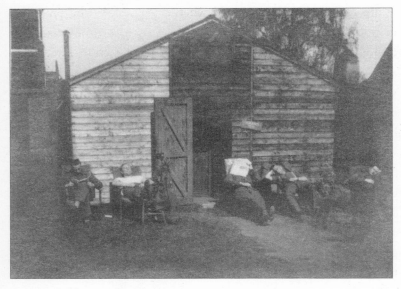

The sergeants hard at it on a Sunday afternoon.

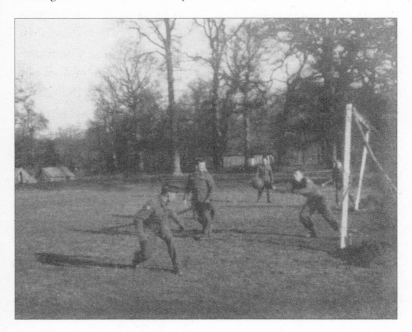

And interdepartmental football knockabout.

No one in the mess minded whether they added up properly or not, but somehow a decent set of figures had to be presented to higher authority. As the furrows disappeared from Paddy's brow and his readiness to take offence where none was intended gave way to comparatively calm normality, we knew that the crisis had passed and a balance had been achieved. Somehow the barrel of beer for which no one seemed to have signed any chits had been written off, somehow the deficiency in stock had been lost in a sea of figures and we could start the month with clear consciences once again.

In our mess it was only some of the padres who seemed ill at ease and out of place. For a Church of England or nonconformist padre a medical unit is probably one of the most difficult appointments to fill successfully. He usually finds himself among officers who, even if not antagonistic to his doctrines, are not enthusiastic in their support, and in a theological argument he may well encounter a doctor more perfect in the factual knowledge of the Bible than he is himself. In the Medical Corps, too, the gap that separates officer from man that is found in a combatant battalion does not exist. Whether lieutenant or captain, major or colonel, the officer still remains a doctor. He still remains a doctor to the other ranks particularly, and because of that many of their troubles are taken to him instead of to the padre. The latter does not have the same position of initial contact that he carries in a non-medical unit and from the start his task is made more difficult.

A continuous stream of Church of England padres passed through the units with which I served. They came, they saw, but I doubt whether they ever conquered in the few months that each remained. To do that required a wider imagination than most possessed. It required a more personal and intimate presentation than the majority were able to give. Religion did not consist alone of services in a tent that had been converted into a House of God.

It lay around the man's bed, mixed with his suffering, in his hopes and often in his despair as, worn out and weary with the struggle against his awful wounds, he more than ever needed the strength and fight that alone might save him. So many of the Church of England padres found themselves in an atmosphere in which they were not at home. It was not their fault. It was grim enough for those of us who were used to it. For them it must have been beyond understanding. There were, of course, many who, in spite of these circumstances, made a difference, offering the sympathy and understanding that the good doctor could offer, but bringing as well the peace and consolation of the gospel. Somehow I think our CCS was unlucky in our Church of England padres for none of them who spent a few months with us were ever loth to leave.

In our nonconformist Church of Scotland padre who joined the unit in Cambridge we were happy because he brought with him less formality and a deeper understanding of all the difficulties which beset us, and when there is this understanding, sympathy and guidance can so much more easily be offered across the ties that have been formed. His name was Dewar Duncan and his Christian integrity was a passport to his acceptance. I do not think he had ever travelled far from the narrow confines of his parish in Forfar, and to be thrown into the deep end in the form of a medical officers' mess and a very experienced RAMC unit must have been a formidable challenge. Our conversation in the mess and our language, too, were certainly not of the kind to which he had been accustomed in the manse. But he accepted it all knowing our only real concern was to continue to lead a medical unit as good as any in the Corps. He helped whenever he could in the preliminary preparation of the CCS and when the time came and casualties began to pour in, he was the only padre who helped with the stretcher bearing and the cleaning up of our theatre. He made a very good cup of tea as well.

A new commanding officer was posted to us. He had served with the cavalry before taking up medicine fairly late in life. We liked him but we soon realised that he was indecisive and lacking in the drive and determination that must be the attributes of any CO, however small the unit he leads. On the reserve of officers, he had been recalled from general practice and his knowledge of the requirements of a unit basically concerned with surgery was not wide. We all had great sympathy for our colonel because he was such a pleasant man and we did our very best to help. He led the unit into France but the command soon became too much for him and he was sent home.

There was much to do in these months of mobilisation. Once again all the equipment of a large forward medical unit, equipment that when complete was enough to fill some forty three-ton lorries, had to be sorted out and issued to the various wards and departments in which it was projected it would be used. Tentage had to be laced together, set up and taken down time after time until all the stiffness of the new canvas had gone out of it and it was supple and easy to work. Then, when it had been camouflaged, it would be packed away ready for use. X-ray equipment, water sterilisers and electric motors all had to be carefully checked so that when finally the day came, there should be no breakdown or hitch. Medical stores and drugs, instruments and splints were packed away under the supervision of the individual sergeant due to be in charge of each ward, so that he would know exactly where they were when they were at last required.

In the Medical Corps there is always room for ingenuity and improvisation, especially in time of war. That it was necessary was in some ways bad, but at the same time, it allowed for creativity in ideas and design. The CCS, for example, was to have two theatres, but there was only one theatre lamp supplied. That our carpenters and electricians could fashion one out of polished tin, soldered together to form a concave mirror that focused the light from its eight bulbs, was a matter of pride to their departments. Moreover, this lamp was good, and so much better than the one supplied, that a second was made and the issued one thrown away.

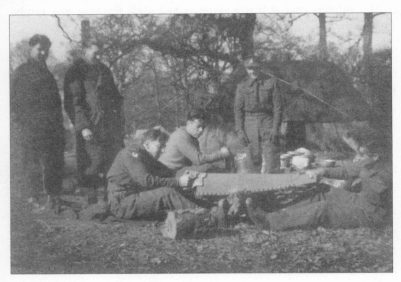

Sawing logs for the cookhouse at Maddingly.

We knew that we should have to take thousands of sterilised dressings with us so that in the first few days of our work we would not be delayed by having to pause while a fresh supply was cut and made ready. The difficulty lay in devising containers in which the dressings would maintain their sterility. Not supplied by the army but made from crude tins rescued from an old dump, our various departments turned out dressing drums that would not have disgraced a London-hospital theatre. These were packed – the smaller with enough dressings to deal with relatively minor wounds, the larger with abdominal sheets and packs and the requirements for any major operation. We took them to the local hospital to be passed through their sterilisers and they were then sealed and stacked with the other operating-theatre equipment ready for loading on to the appropriate lorry when the time came.

It was perhaps because of the scope for imaginative innovation that work in a forward unit offered to the other ranks as well as to the officers that it was a popular job, and one that was rarely filled with anything but enthusiasm. Each ward became very proud of the various improvements and additions it had been able to make to the equipment with which it was issued, and when in practice the wards were assembled, the layout of each was slightly different, representing the ideas of the sister in charge and her nursing orderlies. If something was really required and it was not on the unit's inventory, it became a point of honour that it must be obtained. At first we would ask the quartermaster and, excellent though he was, if you asked him for anything the answer would invariably be no. But, then, with all quartermasters one had learned through the years that their first reaction to any demand was always no. It was second nature with them to refuse, but if you persevered as if you had not heard the blunt refusal, what you required was usually forthcoming.

A typical example was my request for some cases of self-heating tins of soup and Horlicks. I had only recently seen these and I thought how invaluable they might be for our wounded if for some reason, during battle, our kitchens were put out of action. Even a few might help. It only needed the removal of the seal on the underside of the can and the heating mechanism started to work and a hot drink was ready in a few minutes. The automatic no did not prevent my continuing to plead a pressing need for some of these tins. 'I'll see what I can do,' said the quartermaster, relenting, and in a few days a number of cases were there. When he said, 'I'm sorry but I can't help you over that', as he did in the case of the sterile dressing containers, one knew then that a search around Cambridge would have to be made.

About this time I was transferred from the CCS to take command of and to be the surgeon to No. 14 Field Surgical Unit. I was delighted at this. The FSUs, which had their origin in the surgical teams of the BEF, were now equipped with tentage for an operating theatre and a ward of twelve beds, and each carried all its own basic equipment. It had two three-ton lorries and a staff car. The personnel consisted of a surgeon and an anaesthetist, seven nursing orderlies, including a corporal who would act as theatre technician and assistant during operations, and three RASC drivers.

In the forthcoming campaign the plan was that each corps would be served by two casualty clearing stations, to each of which at least one field surgical unit would be attached. Initially both would be opened for casualties, but when the expected advance was about to take place one would close to prepare to follow the divisions involved. The other CCS would remain open to receive casualties up to the very time of the advance and would care for them until all could be removed to a base hospital. It would then close and leapfrog in front of the forward CCS, which in its turn would close, and when its wounded had been evacuated, it would repeat the process.

The FSUs would not stay with the rear CCS but for most of the time would work with whichever one was in front. This plan meant that the FSU would be involved in most of the battles and that its personnel would be utilised with maximum efficiency. In practice, during the rapid advances of the army in France and Germany, the scheme worked smoothly and excellently.

The unit I had joined was by great good fortune to have as its parent the CCS from which I had been posted and which I had temporarily commanded. I had first served with it years before in the BEF and the roots of affection which grow rapidly in wartime were deep. I was glad not to have severed my connection completely.

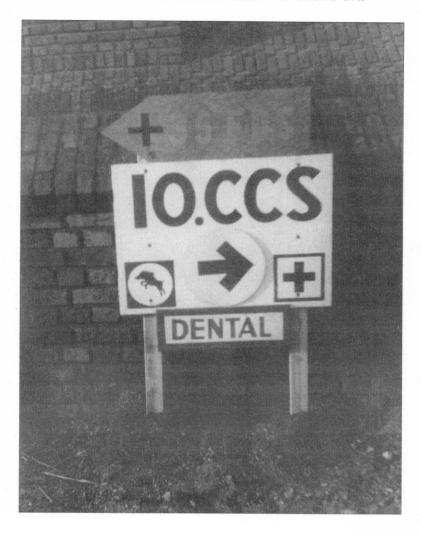

No. 14 Field Surgical Unit was in the process of mobilisation and its equipment was being assembled. The anaesthetist was Major W. Alsop who before the war was on the staff of the Radcliffe Infirmary at Oxford, and he too had recently returned from the Middle East. Apart from his brilliance as an anaesthetist, he was the most delightful of companions. In a small team it is essential

that surgeon and anaesthetist should be able to work together in complete rapport and I knew that this would be so. Moreover, the anaesthetic given to the desperately wounded battle casualty made all the difference between success and failure, the difference between life and death. Its depth had to be exact, not too light so that the surgeon is struggling against contracting muscles, or too deep so that the post-operative recovery of the patient is delayed and his chances of survival thus lessened. With nothing to worry about at the top end of the operating table and the intravenous drips of blood and saline controlled by the good anaesthetist, the surgeon could concentrate his whole attention on his own work.

With the unit were six first-class orderlies and a corporal, Corporal MacGregor, who in civilian life had been an engineer. He was a small Scot but with a large personality that attracted immediate compliance from the other orderlies with regards to his ideas on how his side of the unit should be run. He had been in the St John Ambulance Brigade before the war and had considerable experience working in operating theatres. We knew that this was going to be a first-class unit.

Once again we searched for tins in which to pack our dressings. My aim was to have enough supplies for a hundred operations before we would require replenishments. We found willing helpers in the town to cut the gauze and lint, to sew the operating drapes and to arrange them in the tins, after which they were taken to be sterilised.

Although there were two three-tonners with our unit, an order informed us that only one of the lorries would go over in the first embarkation and the other two vehicles would follow as soon as transport became available. It was therefore essential to eliminate everything but necessities for stowing in the first lorry, and little by little with numerous trials we finally felt that we had achieved the best compromise.

242

I was sent to Salisbury Plain for a few days to talk to the medical side of the airborne division on the treatment of battle casualties. I felt very proud to be among these superb troops, but it became apparent that in the circumstances in which they would find themselves, little treatment more than advanced first aid would be possible. Nevertheless, along with other things I was able to show them the so-called Tobruk method of immobilising fractured lower limbs so that the wounded could be transported with the least pain.

The weeks passed rapidly back at Cambridge. Soon the gold and purple crocus-covered banks and the pale green buds of the willow trees reaching down to an idly flowing river told that winter had passed and another spring was had arrived. It could not be long now before the last act of the war against Nazi Germany began.

We were given a few days leave. I went down to the west of England because in the years that had gone by, in the heat and dust storms of a thousand miles away, I had always had a picture in my mind of a Devon springtime. I wanted to see it once again so that I could take an up-to-date memory back to the life that was war.

There the spring was even more advanced. In banks green with ferns, violets and primroses hid themselves as if afraid to expose their fragility to an unfriendly world. Daffodils were waving in the spring breeze, the buds just coming into bloom. It was exactly like the mirage that had beckoned to me across a waste of sand. The house that I had just left, the sweet fragrance of burning wood, the laughter and tears of children, the sounds of a household at work with all its comings and goings were there at the bottom of the hill.

But I no longer belonged to this scene. Far away nothing had seemed easier than to come back. Now, when the scene lay a few hundred yards distant, there was a chasm of separation, wider by far than the years and the miles. It was a chasm that war had created, which one day peace would bridge. For the present I was more at home in an atmosphere of medical panniers and operating kit, in field units and casualty clearing stations. As I wandered through lanes, high hedged and bursting into leaf, where the air was filled with the fresh smell of good earth moistened with spring showers, as I looked down on the village where the smoke trailed dreamily into the sky from thatched or slated roofs, I knew that I had little part in all this. Here peace and eternity seemed to lie. Here there was no place for doubt or wondering, only an age-long conviction that life goes on. For a few days I had shed my khaki, pretending I could forget the war. But it was not only a different coloured suiting that the army had given me: it had given me a different outlook as well, and in a few brief days this was not so easily put away as the uniform that took but a few moments to hang up in the cupboard.

As May came, the last stages of our preparations were almost complete, and we forward surgeons received a final briefing from our consultant. From our meeting with the brigadier, there must have been few of us who did not come away with some feeling of depression. It appeared that during the first fortnight or so of the invasion, it was unlikely that the Corps, with the limited facilities with which it was to work, would be able to put up enough beds to cope with all the wounded that were expected. In so far as was possible, we were only to deal with the very worst cases and all others were to be evacuated back to England without preliminary surgical treatment. Those with abdominal wounds were to be considered largely in the latter class.

The brigadier knew as we did that his words meant disaster for many wounded men, but there was no alternative. It was quite useless to spend hours operating on a man with a shell or gunshot wound to his abdomen if he could not be skilfully nursed following the operation. The latter was just as vital to his recovery as the former, and if the bed situation was under so much strain he would never receive this aftercare. Although all of us knew how, with each hour of delay, the man's chances of recovery from such a wound became rapidly worse, it seemed that his best hope lay back in England if the nursing that followed his operation in France was going to be so limited. It was a terrible choice to have to make. Both courses of action meant that the soldier who received an injury of this type, from which in normal circumstances he would stand a reasonable chance of recovery, must now be considered as being mortally wounded.

Although every instinct of our medical training revolted against this idea of abandoning a man to his fate, we knew that our surgical brigadier felt the same, and that for once military necessity had to have dominance over what we would have wished. With landing barges and ships at an absolute premium, it was obvious that our requirements should take second place to those of actual battle. It was the price to be paid for invasion, but it was none the less depressing for all that.

Happily, when the invasion did come, casualties were far less heavy than had been expected and by a great effort all the units of the Corps over in France were able to cope with the wounded, so that few were sent back to England that would have been saved by initial treatment before their voyage.

Our last duty was to make sure that the engine of our lorry was efficiently waterproofed. It was going to be impossible for the bigger landing craft to approach right up on to the beach and the vehicles would have to run down the ramps of the ship into water perhaps three or four feet deep. The last fifty or a hundred yards they would have to make under their own steam.

To enable this to be done, every vital part of the engine had to be encased in a plastic asbestos compound and the exhaust pipe had to be extended so that it protruded above the roof of the vehicle. Practice waterproofing was always popular because it was accompanied by a test with the vehicle loaded with troops. Sometimes, in traversing a large expanse of water, an engine would reveal some small fault in its proofing by spluttering to a stop. One vehicle and some twenty men would be marooned to the delight of the onlookers, both civilian and military. But the RASC drivers rapidly mastered the technique so that, while the water whirled about their legs, the lorries could navigate a fairly deep pond with comparative ease.

In the middle of May a bitter blow was dealt to our unit. Major Alsop received an unexpected posting order and was transferred to one of the two-hundred-bedded hospitals which were to be the next to follow the casualty clearing stations in the build up of RAMC services on the Continent. It seemed a most senseless move to have ordered at this very late stage in our preparations, when whoever was sent to take his place could scarcely get to know the unit or be of much help in the packing and loading of our stores. I awaited Major Alsop's replacement with trepidation.

A few days later a young officer joined us and on the morning after his arrival I discussed with him fully the various problems of anaesthesia in battle casualties. I was dismayed by his lack of experience in the anaesthesia of general surgery, let alone that of war casualties, of which he had none. I knew that he was not competent to deal with the work that lay ahead. It was not his fault as he had joined the army and went where he was sent. It was, however, the fault of the consultant anaesthetist who had made the change to my unit. In fairness to myself and to this inexperienced officer, and to the wounded of whom we should soon have responsibility, I decided to go to London to see this consultant.

I explained the position and begged that I be given an anaesthetist of greater experience or, preferably, that Major Alsop should be sent back; but this arrogant man, a senior consultant to a great London teaching hospital, refused to listen to my request.

He had placed the pieces in his little game from his velvet-arsed vantage point and nothing was going to budge them. 'In any case,' he concluded, dismissing me, 'Major Alsop is too old to serve with an FSU.' I laughed hollowly and said, 'In that case, why was he ever appointed?' There was no answer to this impertinence to a senior officer and I left. I went back to Cambridge depressed, knowing that some disaster was bound to overtake my unit and that this fool would be directly responsible.

On 1 June our orders to remove to a concentration area were received. The lorry was loaded and carefully checked and the CCS prepared to move as well. Our own vehicle was filled to overflowing. Beds were laced on to its sides and tents were strapped on to the canvas canopy. There was not a cubic inch to spare and orderlies had to hang on as best they could. It was a very secret move but everyone in Cambridge must have known that the CCS and its attached units were moving out. At zero hour in the early hours of the morning many came to wish us goodbye and a safe return.

We arrived in London as the morning workers were hastening to their jobs. From all parts convoys were streaming in, eventually to cross the City towards the concentration areas near the docks. They formed an endless procession of armoured vehicles, guns, troops, transporters and lorries, mixing with the London traffic, turning the City into an armed camp. Here and there we received a smile and a wave but for the most part there was little sign that this torrent of transport was anything new to London. All understood its purpose; all knew that for some this was their last journey, but too much rested on this enormous project to approach it with anything but humble hope. It was a time for the average Englishman to hide his private thoughts. Only by carrying on as if nothing was afoot could he give what to him was a true expression of his feelings.

We paused short of the East End and moved into a part of the enormous camp at Wanstead. It was heavily wired and guarded. There was only one way out from here – down the Thames and across the Channel. The few days that remained seemed long. Once we had been issued with sealed maps and orders and our money had been changed into unfamiliar French-franc promissory notes, there was little to do. Anxiously we listened to each wireless bulletin, wondering how much longer the suspense would last. The weather seemed not to be in our favour and perhaps because of this there was extra delay.

Then, on 6 June 1944, the news of the invasion bellowed out through the loudspeakers. We knew that we should be leaving that day. In the afternoon we drove through the East End to the docks. Life on the surface was going on as usual on this the greatest day of all. There were crowds in the streets and queues waiting patiently outside the shops. But each heart must have been praying silently and very fervently for someone very dearly loved who had already launched the attack on Hitler's 'Atlantic Wall'.

16

D-DAY AND ITS AFTERMATH

JUNE 1944

Normandy landings, 6 June 1944; CCS set up near Bayeux;
dealing with casualties and an incompetent anaesthetist

We embarked on a Victory boat, the *Fort Norfolk*, and in the darkness we sailed down the Thames to anchor at its mouth until daylight came. Then in a large convoy, guarded by warships, we sailed south towards the Channel.

As we passed through the Straits of Dover, a dark cloud of smoke was laid by the escorting destroyers to blot out the convoy from the eyes of the artillery watching it from Calais. It had been four years since I had seen the convoys running the gauntlet up the Channel, blacked out and protected by smokescreens as they passed through the narrow strip of water. Now I was in one of those convoys but heading west instead of east. Four years ago there had seemed so little chance that one day we would come back, but now the tide was flowing after its ebb and, strong and powerful, we were returning, not alone now but with gigantic allies, buoyed up with the hopes and prayers of all who longed for escape from the darkness.

It was impossible to see or know what was going on with the clouds of smoke billowing out over the sea all around us, but the convoy emerged into the open Channel intact. Gradually behind us the screen of smoke that had protected us faded like a morning mist on the horizon. We went on, now with an added air escort that circled everlastingly around the line of ships it was protecting. Ours was not the only convoy sailing down the Channel on this summer morning; in fact it seemed that from every direction all types of vessel were hastening to a rendezvous. Already enormous blocks of concrete, which were to form the prefabricated harbour on the beaches of Arromanches in Normandy, were underway, bobbing up and down as they were towed gracelessly towards France.

This was the first Wednesday in June. In times of peace, thousands upon thousands of cars would have been converging from all parts of England on the downs at Epsom. Now hundreds upon hundreds of ships carrying just those same people were hurrying to a different meeting, where the stakes were higher, and where the gains and losses were not just pound notes and shillings, but freedom itself or perpetual serfdom.

On the morning following, the huge armada that lay off the beaches of Arromanches ceased to be tiny specks that ridged the sweeping line of the horizon. As steadily we approached to join them, the outlines of battleships and cruisers, merchant ships and landing craft, became distinct and recognisable and within a short time we too were a part of this enormous army of ships.

We anchored half a mile away from the shore. Stretching far away to the west, stretching towards the east and to the north, everywhere there were ships, as if all the vessels of England and America were assembled in these few square miles of sea bordering the coast of France. They might have been awaiting some naval inspection as they lay pulling at their anchor chains and slowly and methodically discharging their cargoes of men and materials onto hundreds of small landing craft that chugged backwards and forwards to the beaches. Only the roar and flame of the navy's guns pouring their shells into German positions far back reminded you that not many miles away an enemy was trying desperately hard to destroy a bridgehead that had been gained so gallantly in the last days.

On the foreshore were the relics of those early hours. Landing barges in their tens, smashed and buckled, lay strewn about the sands, some thrown high up by explosions, others sunk in the shallow water, while bent and twisted girders and shattered concrete blocks marked the gateway that had been forced into the northern coast of Europe. The obstacles were not yet all cleared and unlucky craft and vehicles were still striking hidden mines. But for the most part a safe run-in had been established by the sacrifices of those who had dispelled the myth of an impregnable Atlantic wall.

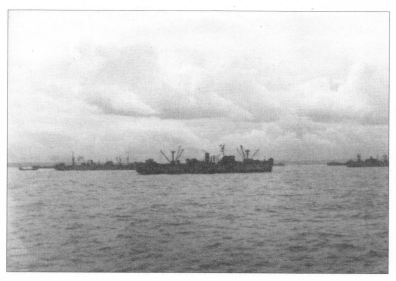

Transports lying off Arromanches soon after D-Day.

Bad weather on the previous day had delayed landing operations and we had hours of waiting, hours that seemed very long because we were anxious to get started on all the work that we knew must be piling up there on the beachhead. I walked up and down the limited deck space until I was tired of walking. I tried to rest but could not. Now and then I leant over the rails scanning the shoreline with its tiny village that looked from the ship so peaceful and unspoiled. It was the illusion of distance. It was the same illusion that had made Tobruk look unspoiled from far away. From over there came the rumble of explosions and now the flash and smoke of bursting shells on the foreshore. No, it was not really peaceful there in that village by the sea.

As the long summer day was fading into night, craft came alongside to disembark us. The many vehicles on the ship were swung up on the derricks and lowered over the side on to the landing craft. I watched anxiously because the men working the donkey engines did not seem to be very expert at their job. With each swing of the derrick they were only just missing the deckhouses, and the vehicles were swinging in dangerous arcs.

At last our precious three-ton lorry started on its journey. It never looked very safe and within a few moments it was swinging backwards and forwards dangerously, scattering troops in all directions and tearing through the deckhouses. From its tightly and carefully packed interior, bandages, dressings and drugs came tumbling out, while its whole superstructure leant over at an ugly angle. There was a large dent in the bonnet; my heart sank. If we could not get the lorry ashore we were comparatively useless, for without his equipment a surgeon can do little.

When the vehicle had at last arrived on the landing craft, we inspected the damage. Fortunately it looked superficial and the waterproofing seemed intact. The loss of drugs and dressings, which had mostly fallen into the sea, we could afford because I knew that we had come plentifully supplied. I had a feeling of great relief that all our hard preparations had not been set at nought before we had even started.

The day had almost passed as we made for the shore. The landing craft was filled with overloaded vehicles, their crews hard put to find a place to perch. All of us were tense and excited. I was glad that ours was not the leading lorry. In a few minutes the ramp of the landing craft would be let down and the leading vehicle would run down into the sea. All would probably be well, but there was just a chance that there would be a dip in the sand there, or a large shell-hole filled with deep water. It was bound to happen occasionally, so I was glad that we were lying second.

The dark shore lay ahead dimly. In the glimmer of fading twilight it looked far away. You could see the silver of the waves breaking on it. The landing craft stopped. The ramp was run down. All the drivers were revving up their engines. We scarcely noticed a cacophony of sound and light from all the ships that were firing madly at the raiders, who only dared appear when night came.

The ramp settled down at an acute angle, meaning that the water must be fairly deep. The front vehicle started and the sea pushed away from its blunt radiator. It dipped as its front wheels left the ramp and fell on to the sand, then roaring wildly it was away. We followed. The ramp was even steeper than it looked and we clung to the roof of the lorry tightly to prevent ourselves skidding off. There was a big bump and we were jerked forwards as the full resistance of the water met the lorry. But the waterproofing was fine and we were soon making for the shore.

Scattered around about were the silhouettes of various armoured vehicles and lorries that had got stuck. We were pleased that our proofing was perfect and shouted excited encouragement to our driver. Suddenly the lorry seemed to collapse and tilted over to one side. We skidded off the roof and into the sea. By bad luck we had driven into a shell hole and the wheels were flying round wildly, unable to get a grip on the soft sand. We knew that the tide was running in fast and that there was little time to get out before the lorry was irretrievably submerged. All our efforts to help by pushing were useless, so I waded ashore to find a salvage unit. Happily I saw a tank coming up out of the sea on to the beach. I shouted to the driver and asked him for a tow and within a few minutes we were lugged out of our hole and were safely on the shore.

It was pitch dark now as we groped our way up the tracks leading from the sands to the road above to join an endless stream of vehicles following each other away from the beachhead. Sitting beside the driver, trying to help him pick his way over the battered road, I heard a voice in my head which kept saying, 'We've come back to France. We've come back.' In the blackness there was little to see. Only the ugly outlines of shattered homes, and they could be seen anywhere across the weary face of Europe. But we were back again. That for the present was enough and I was almost happy. As we went further away from the beaches, the traffic thinned out a little. We tried hard to find the CCS we were to join but no one knew where they were and rather than wander aimlessly, searching in the dark, I decided we should rest for the night. We drew off the road into a field and although wet and cold we slept soundly by the side of the lorry until dawn.

All ranks carried with them concentrated rations, enough for forty-eight hours, and from these we breakfasted, crumbling the oatmeal cake into water and boiling it on our 'Tommy cookers'. It made a very reasonable substitute for porridge, and the mixed powder of tealeaves, dried milk and sugar, which we boiled in water, produced a beverage resembling tea. Even if it only resembled tea, in the cold of the morning with our clothes still very wet, it was warming and delicious.

Soon we located our rendezvous, but the CCS had not yet

arrived. I reported to an administrative office to see whether we could attach ourselves to some other unit until they came, but I was told to wait; it was not until the evening that their advance party turned up. They had been delayed in disembarking.

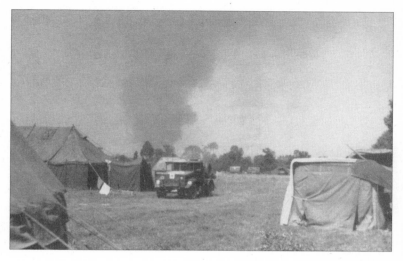

No. 10 CCS at its first location near Bayeux, June 1944.

We moved to a small village a mile from Bayeux to select a site for the unit. We chose a large field and at once started to cut down hedges in order to make a runway in for the ambulances and lorries. We had not been working more than an hour on this job before a Frenchman came up. Apparently he owned the field, and, while welcoming us to France, he wanted to enquire as to whether we were going to use his field, because if so he wished to make a claim for its use. He was certainly a man with a practical turn of mind.

As we finished clearing the hedges, the CCS lorries arrived. Each contained the equipment of one department or ward and was unloaded opposite a corresponding sign that we had pegged into the ground when planning the layout. Experience in the desert and all the months of training since its return to England had made the CCS first class. Within a few hours of its arrival, a bare field had been transformed. Now it was covered with large hospital marquees and smaller tents. Inside were operating theatres and clean white-sheeted beds, laboratories and X-ray units; administrative offices had been set up and tentage for personnel, and tucked away in one corner our cooks were already preparing meals for the wounded troops who were soon to arrive – and to arrive in such numbers that we were in danger of being overwhelmed with casualties.

The ambulances started to pour in during the early hours of the morning, and continued to do so for the next three weeks. On paper the CCS with its attached unit was designed to cater for about a hundred beds and a similar number of stretcher cases. In actual practice, during the early days of the invasion, often more than fifteen hundred wounded passed through the unit in a twenty-four-hour period.

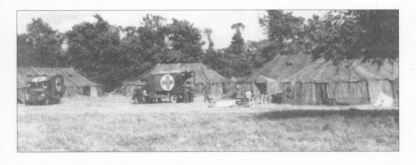

Although we were evacuating all the time to the beachhead evacuation centres, sometimes we were so inundated with casualties that there was literally not a square foot in any of the tents on which to accommodate them and for a while they had to lay on their stretchers in the open. Fortunately, most of these wounded could be sent directly to England, especially as we had in our armamentarium phials containing penicillin. It is to this wonder drug, which was injected into every patient with anything more than superficial wounds, that the prevention of sepsis and the curtailment of the period taken for recovery was largely due. Instead of arriving in England with their wounds stinking with infection because they had not had early surgical treatment, these men returned home in good shape. Few suffered because we were not able to treat them there.

Even though only a small percentage of the wounded required urgent treatment, there were more than enough to keep our pre-operative ward perpetually overcrowded. There was only one way to cope with all these cases and that was to work and work until it was impossible to go on any longer and we had to go away for a few hours to rest and sleep. We were tired, incredibly tired, for the days and nights wore on and still the pre-operative wards were always full. The faces changed from day to day but still there were the same dreadful heart-rending wounds. The shoulder badges of different regiments were there, but the clothes were all equally caked with drying blood and torn and ripped open by high explosives.

The wards and our theatres became our real home during those weeks. Only occasionally would we leave to lie down in exhausted sleep in our own tents or to steal a precious hour in a field nearby, away from the relentless tragedy of it all. But even when you were away you could not really relax because you knew there was so much to do. That for the present was all that mattered.

I do not think that we were very 'normal' mentally at the end of those weeks. Perhaps most of us had been away from the sight of war wounds for too many months, so that we had lost our familiarity with the cruel and terrible atmosphere of pre-operative wards. And suddenly here it was again, overwhelming, worse perhaps than ever before. The legs and arms seemed more mangled and the bones more shattered and more starkly sticking out. There were more faces too that had been transformed into ugly gargoyles, not frightening but so utterly tragic that you had to make an effort to prevent your tears welling up uncontrollably. You wanted to rush out and cry aloud to someone to stop this slaughter that wrecked everything that was lovely and blameless. But you went on, looked at others, saw guts hanging out, with the faeces oozing on to the surface, or perhaps genitals that lay ripped from the scrotum and covered only by a dirty bit of bandage.

Blood was transfused steadily into the veins of all these men as they lay there, mostly only semi-conscious, gaining strength from rest and treatment until they were fit to stand an operation. Most of these poor wounded we knew we would save, and the majority would return to something like normal life. But the man with his testicles torn away, the one blinded in both eyes with an arm that was hanging on by a few shreds of skin and muscle alone, which we should have to take off, or another who was going to have both his legs amputated at the thigh very soon in addition to the treatment of his other wounds, were we right to fight so very hard to save them? Sometimes we wondered, but in spite of all the logic in our hearts we knew we were right, whatever the future held for these terribly maimed men.

In this atmosphere of the pre-operative ward, eerie in the dim light of the night hours, we would gather in-between operations to drink one of the numerous rounds of tea without which we would never have kept going, and to talk about anything in the few minutes before the next patient was prepared on the table. We were ready to laugh at anything, ready to laugh even at death when death was hovering round some of the patients in the ward. Here where men were 'hanging up their saddles and going into the last weighing-in room', we jested and talked. To an outsider we would have sounded callous in the extreme, but we had to find something to laugh at, no matter what it was, else we could not have borne it all.

About ten days after we had returned to France, our sisters arrived. How very happy we were to see them because we knew now that much of the worry of the post-operative nursing of our patients could be left in their very capable hands. Our nursing orderlies, who in their care of these desperate wounds had done more than any of us doctors could have expected of them, were good, but however good, the expertise of a first-class sister was that much better and could make the difference between success and failure. As they arrived at the CCS in their battledress blouses, khaki slacks and boots they did not look like sisters used to. In fact, some of the wounded lying in the open thought they were a party from ENSA come over to entertain them. But we knew who they were and we were very grateful for their coming. In the operating theatre we could get on without them, in fact we were better off probably with first-class RAMC personnel theatre assistants because there was such a lot of heavy work in a forward theatre. However, in the wards it was a different matter. That fine gap between life and death was widened now. We stood a better chance.

In spite of all our efforts, sometimes there were those who disappointingly slipped away from us. We expected them to get better. In the pre-operative ward they responded to treatment, in the theatre it seemed that their wounds, although severe, would heal. For the first few days in the wards they would do well, and then as you watched them you knew that they were losing ground and that you were losing, too. You would renew your efforts, try everything in a last desperate endeavour, but sometimes nothing was of avail, and in those early hours of the morning when life seems at its lowest ebb, they would pass into the great beyond. It seemed as if the body and the mind had become tired of the long struggle and had suddenly given up. Such cases, when everything I suppose was just too much for the frail human body to stand up to and fight against, were depressing and disheartening.

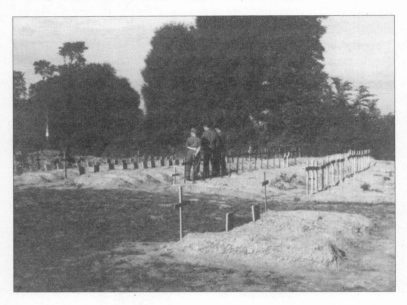

A British cemetery at Bayeux.

One day a patient arrived in the pre-operative ward. He was not terribly wounded and could have travelled on to England without initial treatment, but as he was there we decided that he should remain and we would deal with him in-between more serious cases. He became a bit fed up with waiting because he was very hungry and as he was going to have an anaesthetic we could not allow him to eat anything. Each time one of us was about to take him into the theatre, we saw some more urgent case that we had to deal with first, and so the hours of his waiting grew longer. He was not a cigarette smoker but said that if only someone could provide him with a pipe and tobacco he would be all right and would not mind the long wait. From somewhere these were found and then he was happy, as he sat there, propped up on his stretcher, puffing away while all around were heard the involuntary groans of the badly wounded. Every time a surgeon came out of one of the theatres – there were three running out of the ward – he would put down his pipe and a smile of anticipation that his turn had come would spread over his face. Then as the surgeon passed him by to deal with some more urgent case, he would suck again vigorously at his dying pipe and settle down with a sigh of resignation to a further wait. This happened many times in the twenty hours he had to stay there. But at long last his turn came and with a happy smile he was carried in to have his operation.

In spite of all the work we were doing I was very unhappy with the way things were going in my unit. Too often I was struggling against an anaesthesia that was too light, and too often I felt that a soldier's return to consciousness after his operation was unduly delayed. Some had died and I knew in my heart that two of these deaths could have been avoided. My concern was shared by my orderlies, who were also anxious about what was happening. All the doubts I had expressed to the consultant anaesthetist in London were no longer doubts; what I had warned him about had come to pass. Late one night a Scot lay on the operating table. He had a penetrating wound to his abdomen with early peritonitis. I explained to him what I had to do. 'I know you'll do your best, doc, and I'll be all right.' I had heard so many similar words before. I went to scrub up for the operation and returned to the table. I was about to put on the operating drapes when I realised that the man was dead. We tried desperately to resuscitate him but it was to no avail. His was an anaesthetic death.

I was shocked. I knew that I could never operate with this anaesthetist again. I could not blame him; the blame lay with the pompous arrogant fool who, in spite of advice, had placed him in a position for which, as yet, he had not had adequate training. I kept on remembering the Scot's last words: 'I know you'll do your best and I'll be all right', and tears came to my eyes for the body which still lay on the table. I felt sick and crushed and at the same time very angry that this should have occurred.

I told my corporal to take away the body and to close the theatre. I had decided to go to army headquarters and ask to be relieved of my major's crown so that I could be sent as a battalion medical officer to some fighting unit just as a captain. At least then I would not have the responsibility of soldiers' deaths to weigh on my conscience, which, with my being the CO of the unit, was certainly the case now.

I alerted my driver and as the first streaks of dawn lightened the sky we set out. Eventually we located the camouflaged headquarters. The Assistant Director of Medical Services was not up but he was roused from his bed. Somewhat incoherently I told him what had happened and what I wished to do. He said that he could do nothing and that I would have to see the consultant surgeon, Brigadier Porritt. To him I once again poured out my story, not calmly because I was no longer calm, but my position was fully understood. He knew that I had done my best to prevent tragedies like these by going to see the consultant anaesthetist when I was in London, concerning the young man who had been posted to my unit, and I am sure he thought me worthy of better treatment than I had received. Two cups of tea were sent for.

'You know,' the brigadier said, 'there is no need for you to stop doing surgery. I will post to you any anaesthetist you care to name, provided he is over here in France.'

'Has Major Alsop arrived?' I enquired.

'Yes,' he said.

'Please may I have him.'

'He will be sent today,' was the reply.

I returned happily with my mind at peace. I knew now that

everything would be all right and when I told my orderlies they knew this too.

That afternoon my old friend Bill arrived. It appeared that he had been quietly making himself comfortable in the small hospital to which he had been posted and which only a day or two earlier had arrived in France. He was astonished to receive a message: 'Report forthwith – repeat forthwith – to No. 14 Field Surgical Unit.'

The ambulances were still pouring in and within a short time of Bill's return a sleepless but very happy unit was hard at work again. Now we were completely confident that the very best would be done for the wounded. Even now, many of their faces are as fresh in my memory as if I had seen them only yesterday. I could pick them out from a crowd and yet when I saw them it hadn't been for long, and each face was one among a host of others. The soldier whose hands were in such a mangled mass that for minutes I debated in my mind as to whether I was right to attempt to save them before finally deciding to do so. The man who flew home to England looking so tiny on the stretcher because his two legs were even then being burned in our incinerator. They are all there – row upon row of them, indelibly imprinted, with all the courage on their faces that masked their pain and made light of their suffering.

One lad was under eighteen. For five days he had wandered about half delirious, nursing an arm that now was black and green, evil and swollen with gas gangrene, with the bubbles of gas collecting under the dead skin. He had tousled straw-coloured hair. He smiled because he was alive and he could rest and sleep now. His face was deathly white, but, as the pints of blood ran into the veins of his sound arm, it became rosier and he looked like the overgrown schoolboy that he really was. We took off his arm. With penicillin and other drugs we overcame the toxaemia of his gangrene and he went home cheerfully. He had not been a soldier very long. He did not seem to feel angry or bitter that a few days of fighting had brought disaster to him and robbed him of his arm. He was proud to have been in the army.

Other medical units were coming into France and at last the casualties were diverted and the unit, dealing only with local sick, was given a chance to rest a little, sort itself out, replenish its stores and prepare for the next step. We felt that in spite of our initial difficulties we had come out of this first test satisfactorily. We doubted we would ever be asked to deal with more wounded than had passed through in this first month of the invasion.

Bringing in the casualties, we had had good field ambulances. Those of the 50th Division who had worked up and down the desert in the earlier campaigns could not have been bettered, and others who had not had that practical experience were learning rapidly and becoming almost as expert as their fellows. So much depended on these field ambulances; they worked under the most hazardous conditions, often under shellfire, and by their first-aid treatment of the wounded had made all the difference to the subsequent chances of recovery of many men.

In this brief period of respite we visited the town of Bayeux, which miraculously had escaped serious damage. Its twelfth-century church remained unharmed except for a few smashed windows. The town was full of troops, out of the line for a few precious days. They came to have baths and to be supplied with clean underclothes and socks and they came to buy as much as their few francs would allow. They were learning, too, that cigarettes were as important as francs in the exchange rates of commerce. Bill and I had our first French meal at the Lion d'Or. It was a delicious omelette, with Normandy cheeses and a Loire wine.

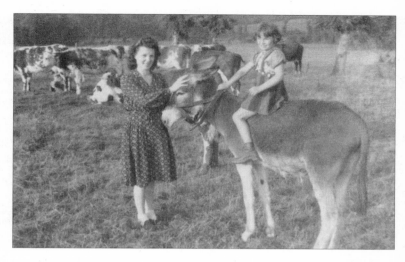

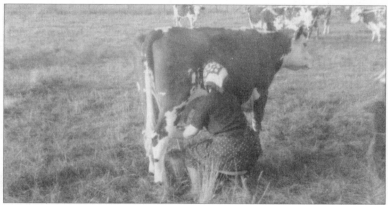

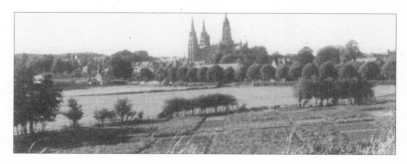

Rural life continued in the Bayeux countryside.

30 June 1944
Major S. O. Aylett, RAMC
14 FSU attached 10 CCS, BWEF

My dear Mum and Dad – A few hours' peace has descended on us and after all the carnage how treasured it is. Death doesn't leave us alone and take a holiday very often. Our resuscitation ward has been filled with groans and grunts and the welling-up of blood and vomit and the despairing sighs of someone passing into Valhalla. I don't think that we have been very normal mentally during the last week. We are apt to laugh when the angels come down with a new pair of wings; we chat glibly in the presence of death. We have to laugh, even though it is hysterical laughter, else we should break down and weep and we could not go on. And so periodically we have our cups of tea surrounded by this atmosphere, find a laugh somehow and at all costs.

The other night we had a patient brought in – he was a German – he was the colour of white paper, pulseless, next to death. He lay on a stretcher breathing with a dreadful gasp about every half-minute. We gave him a shot of morphia and waited for the angels. In between operations I was reviving my flagging body with some tea just by the side of this corpse-like thing when it suddenly sat bolt upright and endeavoured to climb away. God, it was like Lazarus rising from the dead. We were thunderstruck, even awed, and from then on he went right ahead, had his operation and has been sent down the line.

I have seen bad wounds in this war but never so many appalling sights. You would not know some are bodies. It's terrible. I've one chap who is in my ward now who was stinking of gangrene as he lay on his stretcher, his legs just mangled rotting pulp. Now he's better but minus two legs, amputated through the thighs, as well as other awful injuries. Perhaps it would have been better had he died – I don't know. With these very ill patients one is continually fighting, watching them from hour to hour, and after the actual operation trying to stave off the clutching hand. Yesterday five limbs I amputated. I suppose it's bigger and better shells.

Yes, I'd love any periodicals – please send them.

Love,

Stanley

17

THE ADVANCE ACROSS FRANCE AND BELGIUM INTO HOLLAND

JULY–SEPTEMBER 1944

*Keeping up with the advance towards Paris; visit to liberated Paris;
on into Belgium; visit to liberated Brussels; entry into Holland;
attached to CCS at Nijmegen*

By the beginning of July the German armies encircling the British and American bridgehead were starting to give way; 30 Corps had occupied Caen on the 9th and had captured the bridge over the River Orne intact. In the southeast, enemy resistance in and around Aunay was lessening and the town, completely destroyed so that even the roads were unrecognisable, was abandoned on 8 August. The German 7th army lay in a pocket between Falaise and Argentan, where they were to be trapped and decimated.

The war was advancing and No. 10 CCS and my unit were both ordered to close and move nearer the battlegrounds. For the last few days, casualties had been directed to our sister CCS so that but a few patients remained to be evacuated. The leapfrog plan for the two units had commenced, and this short respite had given us time to replenish our packs of dressings, our theatre drapes and stocks of drugs and anaesthetics, ready for the next period of action.

The canvas tents and marquees came down and these and the rest of the vast equipment of the CCS were loaded on to a convoy of some forty lorries. My unit had its own transport, now consisting of two three-tonners and a staff car instead of the single vehicle with which we had landed in France. The field was empty as we moved off, save for one far corner where rows of crosses marked the resting places of those we had been unable to save.

We set up in some meadows outside the village of Balleroy and within a few hours of our arrival we were ready to deal with our first casualties from the battle ahead. The hours and hours we had spent in the desert and in Cambridge practising pitching marquees and tents were paying dividends. Everyone knew exactly what to do and how to do it rapidly and efficiently when setting up or closing down. Which was just as well, for before a week was up we were moving forward again.

On the new site the resources of the unit were once more taxed to the limit. The wounded, both British and German, were brought in by a constant stream of ambulances. The resuscitation ward, erected adjacent to the theatre marquees and communicating with them, was in the charge of one of the blood-transfusion officers, Captain David Muir. Here those so badly wounded that they had to be operated upon were separated from the lightly injured who were moved to the main wards for dressings and subsequent evacuation down the line. Here the blood transfusions were set up. We relied heavily upon Captain Muir in selecting the order in which these dreadfully wounded men should be attended to. There was a limit to the improvement transfusions could make, and if resuscitation was continued beyond that point, the soldier's condition rapidly deteriorated. It was a matter of fine judgement to decide when the opportune moment for surgery had arrived. The canvas corridor which linked the ward to the theatres made it very easy for me and my anaesthetist, or for any of the other surgical teams, to see, in between operations, any wounded man about whom Captain Muir had concerns. Between us we would decide the optimum time for operation. Sometimes I felt that the man would improve if we waited longer, sometimes I knew that he must be next on the list.

Hour after hour we worked. Seldom were we out of our theatre or its adjacent ward, and we often ate where we were. There were snatched hours for sleep and then on again. Our Church of Scotland padre Dewar Duncan helped us, whenever he was free, in whatever way he could. Stretcher bearing, helping to clean the theatre when we had to stop to clear its mess, cutting uniforms off the anaesthetised patients and cleaning the filth and dirt and blood away, and every few hours brewing us cups of tea. It was a far cry from the manse at Forfar but he seemed to have become inured to the sight of abdomens and chests laid open and of limbs being amputated. He was a wonderful help. Our C of E padre – I think we must have had one – I never saw, and our RC one, only when he was administering the last rites to someone already dead or too unconscious to understand a word. One unfortunate incident occurred when Dewar buried a soldier who after the interment was found to have been a Catholic. Soul-searching words were exchanged between the two gentlemen but the ceremony had to be repeated according to the proper rites. No, we were not endeared to denominational religion as we saw it.

We naturally wanted to know what happened to our wounded, whom we never saw again, after they had been evacuated to a base hospital or were back in England. It was important to have this information so that we could judge whether or not our treatment was along the correct lines or whether it should be altered in any way. Forward surgeons in the Middle East had complained of this lack of feedback and the administration of the RAMC had issued us, in this campaign, cards to help us follow up on our patients. On these we wrote our name and unit and the name of the patient. A brief description of the latter's wounds and of his treatment was entered on the card, which, together with the soldier's other documents, accompanied him when he was evacuated. A fair proportion of these cards found their way back to us and on each the final condition of the soldier on his discharge from a base hospital was recorded. The results were more than encouraging and we felt that we could not improve on our present anaesthetic and operating techniques.

Now 30 Corps was beyond Aunay and hastening to help close the Falaise gap. No. 3 CCS advanced in front of us to keep contact, and while No. 10 CCS stayed, my unit left to work with them. The night before moving I wrote a letter home.

29 July
Major S. O. Aylett
14 FSU att. 10 CCS, BLA

Dear Mum and Dad – Thank you for your letter and the cigarettes. Once again we've been worked off our feet and tomorrow my unit up-sticks to move forward and keep contact with the advance. I shall be leaving 10 CCS for a bit and working with another. I think my little unit, which continues happy and satisfied, has done magnificent work. The lads work like Trojans and I have as good an anaesthetist as I have ever met. For myself I feel that I am operating as well as at any time in the past. And yet cases still slip through one's hands, chaps that you think should get better, but somehow they get tired of trying and fade away. I had a lad with a gunshot wound to his tummy. The bullet had gone through stomach, intestines and kidney, and of course an enormous operation was required. He does excellently until suddenly on the sixth day he sits up and *finito* – he's gone. Such happenings, when I suppose everything is just too much for the frail human body, are terribly disheartening and depressing.

The other day I had occasion to go and visit Corps HQ and passed through a small town just taken by the army. I have never seen anything like it – a picture of desolation and destruction compared to which Tobruk looked like a well-built-up area. There wasn't a house standing. Everything was just rubble and a pall of dust hung over the whole town. In parts you could not see the roads; they were hidden by shattered bricks and mortar. Everywhere was the smell of war, acid, poisonous, the smell of death and cordite. The whole aspect of the place was unreal, as if some Hollywood director had ordered a gigantic filmset as a background for some bigger and better war story. Yes, even the dispatch rider was there picking his way through shell and bomb holes, covered with dust, so that his face was ashen grey with it. There is no romance about war, it's just filthy, appalling – only death.

We have lost our old CO and are all very sorry He turned out very excellently, but the powers that be did not think so and sacked him. In his place we have a typical regular. What that means I leave to your imagination. Anyhow, numerous changes in a very excellently functioning unit were put under way. I gently laughed as I had a separate unit and then he dabbles in what is not his business and tells me how to run my own unit. But I've never been much of a 'yes' man and we had a very good row, ending up by his nipping off all lively to the brigadier. I think my stock there is fairly high at the minute, because the CO was just told gently to leave my unit alone. So I hope that will be a lesson to him, but I've been too long in the army to sit down like a junior subaltern and I also do happen to know how to run a FSU.

Love,

Stanley

We worked with No. 3 CCS for several days, operating upon our own soldiers and many Germans, too, who had been brought in from the battle at Falaise. The ring was closing rapidly and the remnants of the Nazi army were escaping through the eastern narrow neck, abandoning all but their lives. The push to the Seine was on and we left to unite with our parent CCS at Gacé. We passed through a once beautiful countryside now spoiled by war. The trees were blasted and splintered. Dead bloated cattle, stinking and covered with flies, shared the fields with German corpses still unburied. The roads were foetid. Mangled vehicles, guns and burned-out tanks – the abandoned equipment of war – were all that remained of the German forces in the gap where they had been trapped.

In the villages on our route the inhabitants were returning to their homes. There seemed to be no resentment that so many of their houses were shattered, that all their personal things, household trinkets, chairs, desks, crockery, wardrobes and dressers lay broken in utter confusion. There was just heartfelt relief that it was all over and the nightmare years had passed. When we stopped these people rushed to welcome us, clung to our hands with cries of 'Mon camarade' and 'Bravo' while tears streamed down their cheeks.

But in some villages there was another sight. Already girls who had cohabited with the Germans were being herded into the square to have their heads shaved by partisans. Somehow there was something especially degrading about this form of punishment,

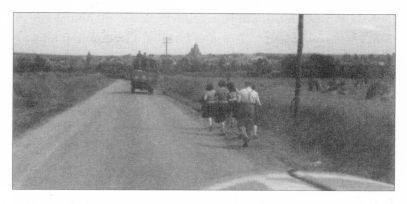

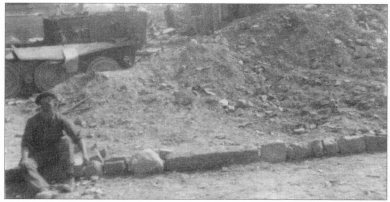

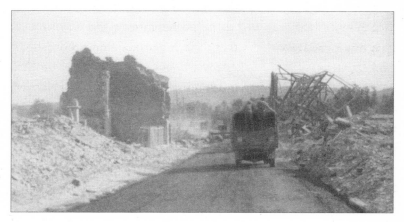

The road through France —Villers–Bocage and Aunay.

both for the women and for those who carried it out, but hatred for the Boche and for all those who had helped him was unbridled.

We rejoined No. 10 CCS a few miles west of Vernon where we were to deal with the flood of casualties likely to result from the crossing of the Seine. The operation, however, was so successful that numbers were relatively small. Resistance on the far side of the river, we learnt, was weak and the Corps was pouring into northern France. No. 3 CCS went ahead and my unit was to be out of action for a few days. We had had no real let-up since our landing at Arromanches and this short period of rest came as a blessed relief.

We knew that Paris, only some fifty miles away, had been liberated a few days before. It seemed a wonderful opportunity to go there, particularly as I was anxious to know what had happened to the French girl from whom I had not heard since I last saw her in Paris in 1940. Transport was no problem as I had my own staff car. This was one of the advantages of serving with a field surgical unit, of infinitely greater value than the few extra pounds I would have earned as a lieutenant-colonel in charge of the surgical division of a hospital, a post which I at one time had been offered. My driver, Lance-Corporal Thomas, was delighted with the idea and early on the morning of 30 August we set off. We took as many rations as we could, as we knew of the shortage of food in the capital.

There were no serious hold-ups on the way and we reached Paris in a few hours. Its outskirts were badly damaged but the centre remained beautiful, exciting and seemingly untouched by war. Everywhere the tricolour flew, often emblazoned with the cross of Lorraine. People rushed to us whenever we stopped, caught us by the arm and embraced us.

'Vous êtes Anglais?'

'Oui, nous sommes Anglais.'

We were the first they had seen for so many years and many faces were drenched with tears.

Yet in spite of the thrill of the liberation it seemed a very weary city, drained by the years of occupation. For weeks there had been virtually no fuel, no oil or gas except for essential services. Food had been so scarce that the black market thrived. Half a crown for an egg, three pounds for a half-kilo of butter. As we drove through the streets we saw that wherever there was a bakery a long queue had already formed. The cafés were shut because there was so little to eat. Here and there a bistro was open serving ersatz coffee and a few drinks.

We made our way to the flat in Montmartre and rang the bell. It was opened by Jeanne's mother, looking a decade older than when I had last seen her. At first she stood back in amazement and then fell against me overcome with emotion. Her daughter was not there but a message was rapidly sent and she came pedalling back on a well-used bicycle. What thoughts surged through our minds – thoughts of years of war, of cruelty, evil and death, and of times when the comfort of brief encounters had saved our sanities.

We spread our rations on the table and a bottle of whisky, too, which we had brought with us. For hours the meal and talk went on; the spam and bully beef had been turned into nothing short of a sumptuous banquet. In the evening we wandered around the city and drank what was called 'coffee' with eau de vie. We stayed in a small hotel that night and early in the morning returned to our unit.

The following day we joined the stream of vehicles of an army advancing. There were hundreds upon hundreds of them of every description. There were transporters carrying tanks, gun carriage after gun carriage, amphibious vehicles, troop carriers by the score, ambulances, lorries loaded with every conceivable item of equipment for war and even the very necessary laundry unit.

The cavalcade rumbled across the pontoon bridge, so brilliantly and recently constructed by the Royal Engineers working under gunfire from the opposite bank. Its every joint seemed to creak and groan under the enormous weight it was being called upon to bear. Yet it was to hold firm for week after week.

Once over the far ramp, we were into the heart of France just south of Les Andelys, where centuries ago Richard Coeur de Lion had built his castle of Gaillard in an endeavour to subjugate the French. They had been liberated from that oppression and now, with the aid of the descendants of those enemies of so long ago, a far more evil overlord of their country was being driven out.

The road ahead led towards Belgium. The villages and towns along our route had not been badly damaged and everywhere their inhabitants lined the decorated roads, cheering, shouting, all so very happy.

We passed through Arras. My mind flew back to that time over four years ago when I had last driven along those same roads. Then I was on the way to Lille and Ypres, a novitiate in the ways of war and in the surgical treatment of battle casualties. I had returned, skilled and tough and tempered like steel in the heat of so many makeshift operating theatres. Nothing could shock or shake me now. No further episodes of war could hurt me as they had. Time was to prove me wrong. Work in a concentration camp was yet to come. Its stark shattering horror lay in the future.

Some miles beyond the town, we opened for a few days. My unit did not unload, as casualties of any great number were not expected and I could use the casualty clearing station's theatres. On 2 September we learned that the Guards Armoured Division had crossed into Belgium through Tournai and on the 3rd they liberated Brussels. I was not going to be operating on the following day and the temptation was too great. We would make a rapid foray into the city along the route taken by the division.

Thomas and I again set off and we soon crossed the border. Every village and town through which we drove was festive with the black, yellow and red of the national flags. They had been hidden or made secretly for this great day and now they flew triumphantly. The streets were lined with people as happy and tear-stained as those in France had been at the news of their release from occupation.

We drove into the centre of the city. The delirious excitement of the past twenty-four hours continued. Our car, marked with the Red Cross, was surrounded. People scrambled on to the bonnet and roof until I thought it would collapse. Flowers were thrust through the windows as we edged slowly forwards. But it was impossible to continue and we had to stop. We were almost dragged from the car. We were covered in kisses until our faces were red with cupid's bows of lipstick. Invitations were poured upon us, to go home, to dine, to have a bath or come to a party in the evening. But we were here for a few hours only and we explained that we wished to wander round the streets and buy a few presents to send home. First, they insisted, we must have a drink and we were escorted to the nearest bar. Brussels was a very different capital from Paris. Here every bistro seemed open and food and drink were available. Perhaps after the first few days of liberation queues would have to form again, but for the moment they were absent.

We finally escaped our wonderful welcome and found a lace shop. We went in and bought several pieces. The two spinster sisters who served us asked whether we would mind coming upstairs to see their very aged mother who was confined to her bed. She, of course, knew of the liberation and had told her daughters that if only she could see a British officer and thank him personally she would ask for nothing more. We gladly went to her room and were introduced to this sweet old lady. Her heartfelt words of thanks and welcome poured out and she gently kissed us both. Now she had contentment and peace and we, for our part, both felt that we had received a blessing, as indeed we had. We made our way back to the centre of the city and were seized and taken to a party. We stayed to drink a toast of friendship, unbreakable and eternal between our two countries, and then returned to our unit.

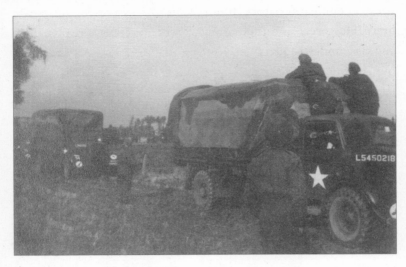

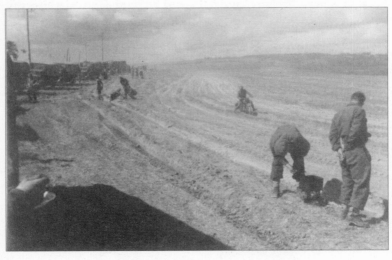

Roadside stop on our journey across France.

The following day we crossed the Belgian border officially. The advance was rapid through the western half of the country and we opened only once. But inevitably the speed of the army's progress slowed. There was heavy enemy resistance in the region of the Albert and Escaut Canals, and near Diest we were again back on familiar territory dealing with torn bodies and shattered limbs. However, on this occasion we were operating in a building and not under canvas. We were spared the labour of setting up our marquees, and for me it was the first time for over a year I had operated anywhere but in a tent. What had been a German officers' mess, rapidly abandoned but with its water and electricity supplies still connected, now served as our casualty clearing station. Although never overstretched, as we had been in the earlier weeks of the campaign, my unit completed twenty-six major operations and many lesser procedures during the three days we were receiving casualties.

Our sister unit went ahead and on this occasion No. 14 FSU was to remain with its parent CCS. We were a little disappointed because a very friendly rivalry existed between the two casualty clearing stations and as we were fully aware the army's entry into Holland was imminent we envied them the honour of the lead into that country.

So we remained for several days looking after our wounded in the wards, evacuating them as soon as their condition allowed and in the evenings sipping Benedictine. When we had arrived in this mess we had anticipated that the German officers would at least have left some wine. But the bottles had all been smashed by the destructive Hun and only a case of Benedictine survived. Even this as an aperitif before our meal of army rations was better than nothing, but since then I have never liked the liqueur.

We were then told that 30 Corps were to spearhead an attack into the very heart of Holland and that we were to be the supporting

CCS, with our destination Nijmegen. We had no hint of Field Marshal Montgomery's incredible plan to establish a bridgehead across the Rhine by means of a combined attack from road and air. That secret was well kept. We knew, however, that this was to be no ordinary advance as our nurses were to follow only after we had reached our objective.

My unit left in front of the CCS and on the 21 September we passed through Eindhoven. Again our welcome was rapturous as the Dutch foresaw the rapid liberation of the whole of their country. Sadly, it was to be many months before that dream became reality.

Our route passed through Oedenrode, some forty-five miles from Nijmegen. The Germans had been forced out of this latter town by the 8th US Airborne Division, with whom the British had linked on 19 September, having fought their way along the road from Eindhoven. But the area on either side of the road from which the Germans had been driven was narrow and it was under shellfire. On several occasions, too, the Boche from east and west were able to link up and to cut off the road completely so that the transport and materials so desperately needed for the relief of Arnhem were held up.

We were stopped at Oedenrode to await our turn to proceed. Vehicles were not now nose to tail but separated by intervals to avoid major accidents should one be hit by a shell. Our turn came to move. 'Keep your feet on the accelerator and your heads down,' we were ordered. Somewhere at the back of the car, hidden under our gear, were our tin hats, but we could not extract them.

We did not have a clear run through. Shelling again halted movement along the road and we left our vehicles to lie in the middle of a field. It seemed safer than in a ditch on the off-chance the Germans had their gunsights trained on target. The field in which we lay was white with mushrooms and when the brief shell storm had passed and its guns had been disabled by counter-fire, we gathered capfuls of these and later cooked them in our Tommy cookers.

I think it had been hoped we would arrive at Nijmegen on the evening of the day of our departure from Eindhoven, but the numerous hold-ups along our route made this impossible. We bivouacked for the night and I chose an unfortunate site for my small unit. It lay by the side of a small wood and in the half-light I had not realised that a battery of gunners had installed themselves there. As soon as darkness fell they started to pound the enemy positions. They continued their good work all night, so we did not sleep.

The following morning came the drone of hundreds and hundreds of planes. We had seen the sky black with a two-thousand-bomber raid when the Germans had been blasted around Falaise and we thought this to was going to be a similar operation. But then we saw they were towing gliders, which when unhooked were gliding into fields ahead of us. A further endeavour was being made to eliminate all enemy forces on either side of the road and to facilitate the attempt to relieve the 1st Airborne Division at Arnhem.

We arrive at Nijmegen on the 23rd after crossing the bridge over the Meuse at Graves, which had been captured intact. The CCS was to occupy a large school sited on a hill below which the Lower Rhine flowed. Here the bridge had also been saved from destruction but it and the town were still being shelled and one of our sergeants was killed.

Again we were quickly ready to receive the casualties from the fighting all around us. Only from Arnhem did they not not come, and it was four or five days before some of the survivors of that great endeavour, exhausted and wounded, were tended by our nurses, who by then had rejoined us.

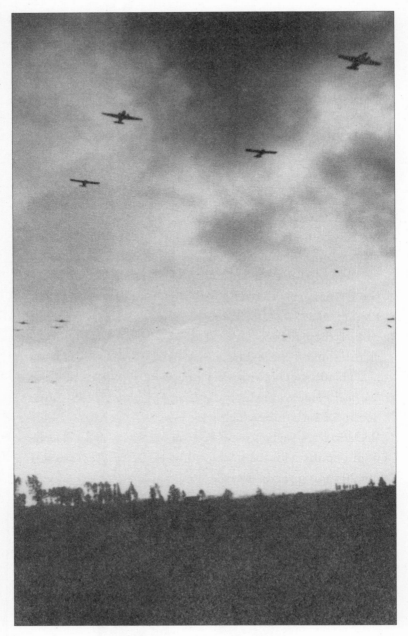

Reinforcements arriving by glider, towed by transport aircraft.

25 September 14 Field Service Unit, attached to 10 CCS, BLF

My dear Mum and Dad,

We have had in the last few days an uncomfortable time but to be part of this gigantic undertaking to cut Holland in half, and split the German army has been well worth it all... .

You must picture to yourself a true spearhead. That is to say that when you're up close to the point and especially if you are the point itself, there are nasty Germans on either side and very close too. It was getting dark then and I hastened to find a suitable field to lodge the unit in for the night. They are not easy to find on account of the ditches and dykes and as I say being near the pointed end it is not advisable to meander far away from the road as little posses of malignant Huns are being continually sorted out from fields not far away. Anyhow, I found what I thought was an ideal field and as it was almost dark, I though how well I'd done. Then as we lined the vehicles round the field there was a noise rather I imagine like a battle ship blowing up accompanied by sheets of flame. We had come to rest at the side of a field containing some dozen 5.5 inch guns which were loosing off at the Germans. Bedlam, I am sorry to say, went on all night, and I was far from popular with the unit, as the guns in some places were not 20 yards from the lorries.

Things became a little unpleasant the next morning and we effected a further small retirement – almost like old times !!!. It was well we did, because not a quarter of an hour after the sky literally became blackened with planes – there were thousands of them, gliders sailed to earth all around. A brief pause followed by a new bedlam of noise, in which the cracking of tommy guns seemed like the tenor in a poor opera company trying to outdo all the others.

Then comes silence and the information that the road is clear – get on a soon as possible. In a quarter of an hour 14 FSU is on the road again, this time going in the right direction. All around are crowds of husky looking American airborne boys, laden with all sorts of instruments of death and destruction.

We come to a town farther up. Once again we are well in the van(guard). We stop at a traffic control post and ask is the road all right. "Well we haven't closed it" is the reply, "it's a bit stick half a mile up, but keep your foot on the accelerator and your head down". So off we go. It's times like this that you wish you could find your tin hat, but of course it's somewhere deep down at the bottom of a pile of luggage and quite impossible to get at. So a gentle prayer to the powers that be, and an adopted air which you hope implies that this is a mere nothing and that of course frightened is the last word you're thinking of, but which no doubt fails miserably – is the best that can be done...

From what I see, and from what I am told, it is impossible to praise the Americans too highly. They are first class tough troops with no-one of the false blah and lack of modesty with which they are normally painted.

There was a battery of guns on the road. They had been attacked and had lost six killed. They decided to go out and see what they could do in the woods at the side of the road. But gunners are ill equipped for this sort of battle. At this moment along came a Jeep with a trailer with Americans hanging on all over the place – they always travel like that. They stopped at the sight of these lads starting to go out 'Say, it's being kinda rough here, is it?' says their commander. On begin told the position 'Okay, we'll fix it. Ed take your gang to the right. Tex, beat 'em up on the left. I'll go in the centre.' Off they apparently disappeared into the woods. For some 20 minutes the gunners listened and all was silent. Then hell's let loose for some 10 minutes, and then after another period of quiet back come the Yanks with many prisoners, having wiped out the rest. 'It'll be okay now,' says their commander laconically...

We are working now in a converted school and it is grand to be in a building once again. I hope that we've done with tents now that we shall be operating in the near future in the Fatherland and can kick a few fat bottoms out of palatial buildings. You can never keep clean, and that does make a difference to doctoring, in tents when the weather is starting to become wintery and wet. The supreme delight of a reasonable building is of course a hot bath.

I hope the letter gets through to Lucienne [the Parisian actress with whom my father fell in love in 1940 and went to find as soon as Paris was liberated]. This time, for all time, I shall get married as soon as I can. You may wonder at all the vagaries of your younger son's 'non-professional' life, but war is a disturbing and unnatural existence and it is easy to have made mistakes that I have made. There will be no mistakes this time.

My love to you. I must go to bed. Stanley

18

ENTRY INTO GERMANY

SEPTEMBER 1944–MARCH 1945

*On to Eisden then return to Nijmegen; posted to join a
Canadian CCS over the border in Germany; rejoining No. 10
CCS at Schloss Wissen; crossing of the Rhine*

We were at Nijmegen for many weeks. Although there was no hope now that the war would end by Christmas and no prospect of the final invasion of the Reich until a new year had come, the German forces were constantly harassed and as a result we were occupied with a continuous, though never overwhelming, flow of casualties. In the school we had all the facilities and comforts we required for our wounded and because of this we were able to keep them longer before their evacuation.

Except for walks in the woods around us we seldom went out of the school and its grounds because of the sporadic shelling of the town. On a rare occasion a friend of mine, a medical officer in the RAF, came to stay for a few nights. He was most anxious to go down to the bridge across the Waal to take some photographs. I was very much against this enterprise but eventually agreed to go with him. No sooner was he poised, ready with his camera, than a shell landed not far away and we quickly abandoned the photography. To court disaster was something I had not done before and would not do again. If we were wounded or killed in the course of our duties, so be it, but to invite unnecessary injury was folly.

In November we were relieved by No. 3 CCS and went to Eisden in Belgium, just west of the Netherlands border. Again we were housed in a school, the largest in this mining town. In the two months we were there we operated upon a hundred and forty-six battle casualties of a major type. Here I saw my first German civilian casualties. They were a girl and a boy, both aged about ten, she with a gaping wound in her chest and he with severe burns and other injuries. After their operations they were with us for a long time but both recovered. 'Is it heresy,' I wrote to my parents, telling them about these children, 'to say that both are so endearing and charming with their happy radiant smiles as they get better that I think I could care for them almost as much as one day I will care for my own? What has happened that their older brothers – yes, and sisters too – may have turned into the beasts of Nazism?'

Social life outside our mess at Eisden was minimal. An occasional beer at some café and that was all. Sometimes we would go to Brussels for the day, as it was only some seventy miles away. There we would always visit the Blood Transfusion Centre to see our friend Colonel Buttle and his colleagues and to discuss any problems that may have arisen. The service we received, however, was so good that it was rare we had any difficulties.

There was little privacy about our lives in the CCS, as all its officers and others attached to it, with the exception of the colonel, slept in a large hall. It was never easy, throughout the whole of the war, to find some place of solitude in which to read and write,

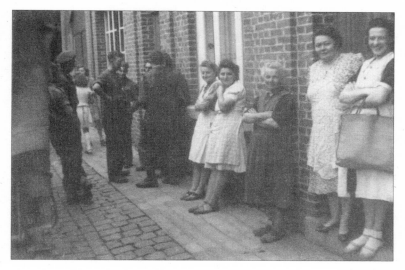

The women of Eisden lined up for a photograph.

to think and to dream. Like a religious community, we lived a communal life, and for us there was not the monastic cell for which, perhaps, we sometimes longed.

10 December, 14 Field Service Unit, attached to 10 CCS, BLF

My dear Mum and Dad,

Firstly I know that you will be delighted to have these two photographs both exactly like Lucienne, the first all dressed up and ready to go out to dinner and the second looking just as charming and all prepared to stay at home. They will give you a little more idea of your daughter-in-law. [My father's marriage to Lucienne had taken place in Paris, 26 October 1944.]

I had a few more lovely days in the big city... Prices are terrific there and there is no doubt that inflation is steadily gaining an upper hand. To eat at any restaurant is prohibitive and to have a good dinner costs about £4 (that's for one person). The smallest, straight forward blouse will cost about £5, or a pair of good shoes £20 or more. I understand from my friends' wives letters that little by little the same thing is happening in England though to a lesser extent. The world seems to have gone completely haywire, and I cannot see any hope of it improving for many years after the war. It is in a sorry state.

Then again the affairs in Greece and Italy with open rupture between ourselves and the Americans. I do not know all the pros and cons of the argument, but surely in time of war suitable negotiation could have prevented this split of opinion. One has a horrid feeling that behind the scenes are many political machinations that have as their object the struggle for power and political domination after the war, rather than the pursuance of the present conflict. It is all rather disheartening...

I and Bill (Allsop) have recently written an article so we hope to get that printed in the next few months. It is on gun shot wounds of the abdomen upon which subject we rather set ourselves up as authorities! It certainly has provided something for us to do...

A year ago today we were sailing up the Clyde. A year filled with great events both personal and general. I suppose we have made great advances, and yet each one of us I think is a little disappointed. May the next few months pass rapidly to victory. There are so many lovely things to be done, so much that is beaautiful and yet all bit by bit is being thrown steadily and surely away. Each passing month destroys and destroys forever and always. There can be no rebuilding of that destruction.

Lucienne has a lovely voice. When we come to London you will hear her.

The post is just going.

On 16 December we heard of the German breakthrough south of us in the Ardennes. There was depression in the town and indeed among us too. We had no knowledge of what resources remained to Hitler, what further fiendish destructive weapons his scientists might have invented. We had seen the pilotless aircraft streaming across the sky towards London, and as some, whose engines had failed, had crashed near to us we were well aware of the devastation they could cause. Was there to be some new and more awful instrument of war that would delay its end after all the hard-fought battles? Fortunately, no surprise 'secret weapon' was forthcoming and by combined Anglo-American efforts the offensive was contained. It was to take weeks of continued battle, towards the end in bitter winter weather, to force the final German withdrawal, but their drive to split the Allied armies and to occupy Antwerp had failed. The cost was many thousands killed and wounded.

At the beginning of February my unit left No. 10 CCS to join No. 3 back at Nijmegen. The push to eliminate all German forces east of the Rhine was about to begin, and we and another field surgical unit were to help in dealing with the inevitable casualties. The CCS, occupying the school we had been in before was in the midst of an enormous army. No one could have blamed the Boche if we had been bombed or shelled out of existence. But now he did not have that capacity; it was only the Allies who had the means to wage a 'blitzkrieg' war. Surrounding us were batteries of guns, some not fifty yards away and actually in the grounds of our building. They were of every type and of all calibres: heavy monsters, seventeen- and twenty-five-pounders, ack-ack guns and Bofors (40mm guns) too.

The CCS was ready and waiting. Its clean beds were empty. It reminded me of the days immediately before the outbreak of war when, at King's College Hospital, the beds were all neat, white and tidy and ready for patients. Our theatres were prepared. We had packed and sterilised thousands of gauze swabs and dozens and dozens of drapes. We had boxes of phials of penicillin and enough Pentothal and other anaesthetics to last for about ten days. There would be no need to halt while further supplies were sent for. Even the first set of operating instruments was boiled and sterilised ready to use. Our blood-transfusion officer was with us, and outside, in a refrigerated van, were the bottles of blood awaiting use in the resuscitation ward. There was no more we could do and we waited tense with the excitement that we were to play our part in this final scene – the invasion of the very Reich itself.

In the early hours of Thursday, 8 February, we were almost blasted out of our camp beds by a violent eruption of noise, as if a dozen thunderstorms had broken around us. We rushed outside. Flashes and flames and belching smoke poured from the gun barrels about us. The night was ablaze with light and on every side were the figures of gunners loading round after round into the breeches of their weapons. We were seeing the biggest cannonade ever fired in the history of the British Army, a cannonade from over twelve hundred guns.

The dawn came and then the daylight, dimming the flashes, but the constant cacophony continued undiminished for about five hours. We wondered how any form of life could have survived this terrible bombardment.

It was the early afternoon before the first ambulances arrived, but happily not in the number we had anticipated the previous day. We knew that somewhere beyond us were fields of mines, which would so readily blow a soldier's legs to tattered remnants, but for some reason these had not been exploded by the shelling. There were also desperately defending Germans who had somehow come through the holocaust of the past night.

I think that our FSU was considered to be one of the most experienced in battle surgery and for that reason many of the most cruelly wounded were directed to us by our resuscitation and blood-transfusion officer. Each wounded man was lifted on to the operating table on the stretcher on which he had arrived in the ambulance. Only when he had been anaesthetised did we take off his clothes and superficially clean him. It would have been too excruciatingly painful to do this while he was conscious.

There was a woman war artist working with the CCS, aged about forty. Bravely she watched us carry out the stages of several amputations, sketching all the time. Then she saw a desperate operation. A fragment of shell had torn a hole through a soldier's right chest wall, lacerating his lung, liver, kidney and intestines. To try and save him was a hopeless exercise but the attempt had to be made. At the end I thought we might have succeeded but he died as the final bandages were being wrapped around him.

Any death on the operating table is a harrowing experience, even when the patient plainly has so little chance of survival. Questions rush through the surgeon's mind: 'Would it have been better if I had just cobbled up the holes in the intestines and thus saved time, instead of suturing them meticulously? Should I have packed the liver and hoped that it would stop the bleeding instead of under-running each vessel pouring blood? Would it have been better if I had simply brought the ends of the severed intestine on to the surface of the abdomen, thus lessening still more the duration of the operation, when speed is so essential for survival?'

For the anaesthetist, too, it is equally distressing. He also has taken this precarious life into his hands. He, with his years of experience, has done his best to give the exact amount of Pentothal and other anaesthetics in balancing the strength between that which the gravely wounded soldier can tolerate and that which will deliver the muscular relaxation he must provide if the surgeon is to be able to carry out his task. He, after a death on the table, agonises like the surgeon.

But when we stood in silent tribute to this soldier as, covered with a Union Jack, he was borne away, I felt that, although all my unit's efforts had been in vain, we could have done nothing more to save his life. Mercifully, there were to be other forlorn hopes that, as some had done in the past, turned to triumphs. It was these that justified our endeavours and salved our aching hearts.

We worked on and the days and nights passed. Then the number of wounded diminished and we guessed that No. 10 CCS had moved ahead and expected to be called to join them. Instead, we received on 3 March an order to proceed at once to No. 3 Canadian CCS where the pressure of casualties was such that further assistance was required. This Dominion unit was operating at Bedburg across the Dutch border, some fifteen miles into Germany.

No urging was required. Our theatre was quickly dismantled and packed. It and all the other equipment of the unit, beds, mattresses, blankets, sheets and other ward requirements, and rations too, were loaded into our two three-ton lorries and into the staff car. We left less than two hours after we had received our movement order.

We crossed into Germany along the road that edged the Reichswald Forest. Only the remains of splintered signs written in German told us where we were. Our spirits were very high. The end of the long years could not be far away now. Five of them had passed since we had expected it to be but a few months before we were 'hanging out the washing on the Siegfried Line', and we had travelled some 10,000 miles to arrive at this final objective. We had a feeling of triumph.

There were towns and villages along our route, or at least what remained of them. Eight months ago the rubble had been French. Now the piles of bricks and mortar which had once been houses were German and it did not seem to matter so much. As my corporal, surveying the ruins of Cleve, said, 'Just the job!' He had lost his home to enemy action.

There were no flags flying here, but where some house stood, still sufficiently undamaged to provide shelter, white sheets of surrender hung and billowed like sails in the wind. Any people that there were lay low indoors, and only a scampering figure suggested that there was still life in the town.

The Canadian CCS was housed in a building of which a large part had been badly damaged, so the rooms which could be used were not many. But being in a building of any kind was better than operating upon and nursing wounded men under canvas in the cold winter weather. The marquees of an established base hospital could be heated readily with slow combustion stoves, but a unit constantly on the move could not provide this amenity.

The colonel welcomed us, I think with relief, as his own surgeons could not cope with the number of casualties awaiting attention. He apologised for the fact that the only suitable space he could offer us was a lavatory, and not an overly large one at that. But I did not mind. The operating table would fit into it and there was a built-in seat for Bill from which he could control the anaesthesia. There would be just room on either side of the table for me and my assistant and we could set up our sterilisers and stores in the corridor from which the lavatory led. It had an advantage, too, in being close to the resuscitation ward, and as Captain Muir was not with us, the selection of the order of cases was largely mine.

We took a little time to make our preparations and in our first session we operated for seventeen hours with only the occasional short break. Then we snatched a brief and exhausted sleep. A few hours later and we were back in our theatre. This was our routine for the three days and nights during which we had the privilege of helping our Canadian friends. Sometimes their nursing orderlies came to see the strange British set-up and one, smiling with

Serial No. in A. & D. Book	Naval, Army or R.A.F. No.	Rank or Rating	NAME (Block Capitals) Surname and Initials	DIAGNOSIS	Date of Operation	Ward	ANÆSTHETIC used and Anæsthetist's Notes
363.	127425	Cpl.	WEST A.J.	Mine. Traum: Amp. R.Leg	9.2.45.		Pentothal.
4.	497343	Sgt.	KELLY	" " " "	"		"
5	2977513	C.S.M.	ENGELS T	" " " "	"		"
6	6108303	Pte.	SMITH B.	2 TST. Pen: G.S.W. Abdomen " Lt Thigh	"	D	" 1.8 grs.
							pr: time. 30.
							died 7 hrs after op: without regaining consciousness
7	0.57593	Pte.	LAPLAINE. A.,	Mult: Mine Wds:	"		
8	14401637	Tpr.	MARTIN J.H.	S.W: Buttocks & Lt Hand	"		"
369	4773375	Pte.	YARNALL C.A.	S.W Abdomen (pen:)	10.2	D	0.8 grs

amusement, particularly at Bill enthroned on his seat, said, 'Well, we've seen everything now.'

It was easier, I had always found, to operate quickly where ample space was available and here this was certainly not the case. Nevertheless, in spite of our cramped conditions, the rows of wounded lying on their stretchers awaiting operation became steadily shorter. Many very major operations were carried out in that lavatory.

The essential details of each patient, of his wounds and the procedure adopted for his surgical treatment, were, as always, entered into our army operating book, and the following are typical of some of those with whom we dealt in this uniquely sited operating theatre.

Army No. B. 116652. Pte Allan, H. M. Injury: Gunshot wound of right thigh, with gangrene. Operation: Amputation through upper third of femur.

Pages from the author's operating logbook.

Army No. 269498. Lt Jones, S. Injury: Gunshot wound of abdomen; bowel protruding through wound. Operation: Abdomen opened; much faecal contamination swabbed away. Large rent in splenic flexure of colon temporarily closed to prevent further leakage. Colon mobilised and damaged gut excised. Transverse and pelvic colon sutured together (Paul Mikulitz-type operation) and ends exteriorised. Operation time 1 hour 10 minutes.

Army No. F35012. Pte Sampson, B. S. Injury: Gunshot wound of abdomen. Operation: Abdomen opened; gross peritonitis; rent of upper part of rectum oversewn; left iliac colostomy formed. Operating time 50 minutes.

Army No. A23331. Pte Newcombe, C. E. Injury: Gross wounds of legs. Operation: Amputation through lower third of left leg; excision of wounds of right thigh.

Army No. 144970. Tpr Maracle, J. R. Injury: Gunshot wound of abdomen; bowel protruding. Operation: Abdomen opened and found full of blood; bleeding points secured; large rent in lower pelvic colon and further one in rectum oversewn. Two rents in small intestine oversewn and pelvic colon brought out as a colostomy. Operation time 1 hour. Patient died in ward.

Army No. 2703004. Gdsmn Garbett, H. Injury: Gunshot wounds of legs and right arm. Operation: Amputation of left leg and right arm.

We were operating on the morning of 6 March and were just completing an amputation through the leg when a message was delivered ordering us to report forthwith to No. 10 CCS at Weeze on the River Niers. The theatre was dismantled, our lorries loaded once again, and after brief farewells to our Canadian friends, we were on the road. I was beginning to think that my unit should be renamed the No. 14 Travelling Surgical Club. We passed through the ruins of Goch and that same evening, with our theatre reassembled, we were operating with our parent CCS. We were to be at Weeze for the next five days.

The German armies were withdrawing rapidly to the east bank of the Rhine, destroying bridges as they went. It was the crossing of this great river, over a quarter of a mile in breadth, which was to present the last major obstacle to the complete defeat and occupation of Western Germany. The operation involved in achieving this aim was aptly named 'Operation Plunder'. Certain amphibious vehicles could cross under their own power and some tanks could be transported in mechanised barges. But for the bulk of the Corps and its associated divisions pontoon bridges were essential. It was the task of the Royal Engineers, one which was to be incredibly performed under constant enemy harassment, to construct these, and of the artillery and other units of the Corps to afford them protection. The CCS was to move forward to receive the casualties from this operation, but while it was closed for a few days so that it could evacuate its wounded and prepare for the next phase of action, my unit returned along the route we had taken from Bedburg to help another to which casualties were being sent.

Four days later we were off again to rejoin No. 10 CCS. A map reference had been given to me and I was told that I would find them in a castle called Schloss Wissen. The prospect of a *schloss* (castle) to work in seemed certainly preferable to the derelict buildings which had been our lot in the last weeks, but *schloss* was a kind of generic word often applied to any house somewhat larger than a semi-detached, so we were not expecting anything special. What the castle was really like and what it held in store for us we could not imagine.

We crossed the Niers over a newly constructed Bailey bridge at Goch. There were refugees on the roads and at one point a large compound for their accommodation had been hastily erected. We had no idea as to what nationality they were, where they had come from or where they were going. They huddled in groups, dejected, unsmiling and lost and we thought they must be German. We continued west following the map. The countryside was relatively unspoiled except for the burned-out tanks and wrecked German guns that littered the roadsides. Quite suddenly we saw the castle to our left. It was incredibly beautiful. The warm rose brick of which it was built glowed in the afternoon sunshine and, by reflection, made red the dark water of the moat surrounding it. Round towers at the corners with blue, slated roofs made the schloss like an illustration from one of my childhood fairy tale books, and a wooden drawbridge connecting it to the surrounding land completed the picture.

Some hundred yards away was a row of small cottages where the workers on the estate must at one time have lived, until the war had taken them away. There were greenhouses and walled kitchen gardens now untended and overgrown. We could scarcely believe that fortune had brought us to this lovely peaceful place, which somehow the war had hardly touched.

We drove to the bridge and were met by some of our fellow officers of the CCS that had arrived the previous day. We asked about the castle and were told that it belonged to a Countess Lowe. She had been living there with two or three elderly retainers when some of 30 Corps' divisional troops had arrived and decided that it was a very suitable place to set up their headquarters. The countess had been told to remove herself and her servants into one of the cottages where she was to stay. Reluctantly, she had consented to obey this order, but on several occasions had been seen in the schloss.

The CO of the troops who were about to leave when No. 10 CCS arrived had mentioned this to our own colonel and suggested that an eye should be kept on the countess as he did not know what mischief she was contemplating. The castle was filled with treasures and the departing unit were taking their share of 'souvenirs', but that, our colonel was assured, there were plenty left to satisfy all – the CCS had no need to worry.

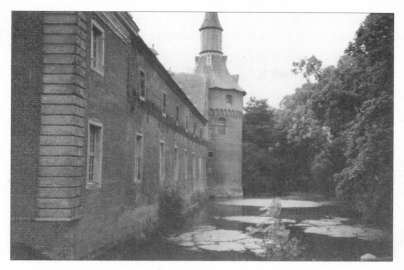

Schloss Wissen near Weese in the Lower Rhine.

A large room adjacent to the main hall, which itself would be used for a resuscitation ward, had been allocated to us and another field surgical unit, temporarily attached to the CCS, as our operating theatre. It was panelled with oak and hung with paintings. We unloaded and arranged our equipment. The schloss was old and unmodernised, with few water points, which meant water had to be carried in buckets from a tap in the pantries quite far away. But the journeys to collect it were well worthwhile because we saw shelf after shelf filled with home-bottled fruits of all varieties and, in a cellar leading from the pantries, found bottles of Rhine wine. We looked forward to these additions to our army rations.

When all was ready, Bill and I chose a room in one of the cottages and laid out our camp beds and our few possessions. Soon the ambulances arrived and the brief period of tranquillity and peace was over. Once again we surveyed the all-too-familiar scene of shattered bodies, guts spewed out, legs and arms blown off, broken bones protruding and faces disfigured – the price these men had paid for building a bridge and crossing the Rhine.

18 March 14 Field Service Unit , 10 CCS, BLF

Dear Mum and Dad,

We are in a castle [Schloss Wissen] – yes. And surrounding it all is a deep moat. It has many turrets and gables, winding staircases that go round and round into the battlements. There are masses of rooms of all shapes and sizes and of course it is quite unsuitable for a CCS, but buildings are few and far between, and although many windows of this one are out and the roof is knocked about it is comparatively intact.

It belongs to an old aristocratic family, the father of whom is now busy pushing up the daisies on the western front, and the son, an SS lad performing a similar function somewhere in Normandy. The widow was living here with her family retainees and on arrival of the CCS she was given an hour and a half to pack what belongings she wanted and to clear out.

A crowd of lads then descended on her home. Imagine all the rooms with masses of furniture, lovely pictures, china and glass. Within five hours it has to be ready to receive patients with the result that there can be no tender handling of the furnishing. The space has just got to be cleared and quickly too.

Fine tables, beautiful chairs, carpets and cushions (she had obviously not responded to Adolph's request for all essential furnishings) go tumbling down the stairs. The more immovable objects go out of the windows into the moat. With little ceremony a fine life-size bust of Kaiser Wilhelm follows suit, with great cheers as it takes a dive into the water... incidentally the count, before he went off to war, was kind enough to leave a very pleasant cellar behind him!

This is what occupation by an army means – something that England fortunately has escaped. There is no longer any right of property. It belongs to the conqueror. I should think the countess must view the wreckage of her home, proceeding before her eyes from the workman's cottage she now occupies, with the feeling that her whole life has been torn apart. It is right that thus it should be.

There is a library of old books, many very valuable, but in one compartment there is tome after tome devoted to war, its prosecution, its art and its science, going way back into the 18th century. These people have lived and fed on war. Now they are going to die and starve on it.

So it went on until the end of March when, a bridgehead established, once again 30 Corps surged forwards, this time towards Bremen. Our CCS stopped admitting casualties and on this occasion my unit remained with them. Our work was now confined to looking after those upon whom we had operated until they were fit enough to be evacuated, whereupon we too could cross the river.

There was plenty of time in which to explore the rambling schloss and its abundant treasures. Old cut glass, rare first editions for the bibliophile, prints and old maps of centuries past, many of them English, were carefully packed to be sent through the Army Post Office to our homes in the United Kingdom. We had no compunction about taking what we wished. Most of us had lost too much as the result of the war Germany had inflicted on Europe not to seize the opportunity of recovering something.

Somewhere in this huge castle we felt sure shotguns, cameras and binoculars must be hidden away. The search went on for these but we could not find them. One of our most enterprising officers took out a boat and rowed around the schloss mapping out a ground plan of the building as he did so. He came back to tell us that he was convinced there was a large area underneath the chapel for which our inside explorations had not accounted. Perhaps it was here that the castle's real valuables were hidden. No entry to it could be discovered in the basements, so we decided that access must lie through the chapel floor above. There no way in could be found until we moved the altar; hidden under this was a trapdoor. Steps led down to a vast cellar on the shelves of which were dozens and dozens of packing cases. We opened some of them but they were filled with sheets and blankets and crockery. It would have been impossible to open them all. Possibly the unit in the castle before the CCS had arrived had found the guns and they were now across the Rhine.

A few days later some members of the military governorate arrived. A decree issued to the German civilian population had demanded the surrender of all weapons, binoculars and cameras; failure to comply with this order could be punishable by death, though I never heard of this final penalty being imposed. Nevertheless, the countess was summoned to appear before these gentlemen and interrogated about such possessions. At first she denied their existence, but when her attention was drawn to the penalty she could incur if a search of the castle revealed any of the prohibited articles, she retracted. The officers were led to the chapel and asked to move the altar. The trapdoor was lifted and they descended into the cellar where the countess pointed to some packing cases on the far shelves. These were opened and there were the forbidden articles for which we had searched. We had been unlucky in opening those close at hand containing only household goods.

Before this incident had occurred, our unwilling hostess had been observed leaving the castle in the early hours of the morning and a watch was put upon her. From time to time she was seen to leave the cottage, slip over the drawbridge and enter the castle through a small door we had scarcely noticed. When she left after a very few minutes, she locked this behind her. Our regimental sergeant-major was soon told of this and a key was found to fit the lock. It led into a room in the centre of which stood a tailor's dummy clothed in an Uhlan general's uniform. Over the left breast was a ragged tear around which was the stain of very old blood. The helmet, too, had a jagged hole. It was the uniform of the countess's husband, killed in the First World War, and it was to this she made her macabre and regular pilgrimages.

The CCS prepared to leave the castle and cross to the eastern side of the Rhine. Several three-tonners additional to those with which it had arrived were required for its transport. The war was obviously nearing its end and all the messes of the unit had rightly decided that wherever it was to be stationed finally, they would live in as reasonable comfort as was possible. We had all had enough of the rough life. Chairs, tables, cutlery and crockery were therefore removed and loaded. The officers' mess had selected a very large carpet and a small Aga-type stove, which we thought would not only keep us warm but would also be the source of meals better than the constant stews and hashed-up army rations of which we were heartily sick. The countess was at the door of her cottage observing with fury the loading of the vehicles. We gave her a cheer and a V-sign as we left.

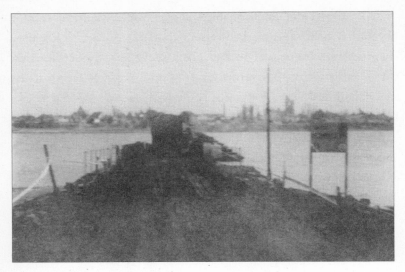

Crossing the Rhine at Rees, North Rhine-Westphalia.

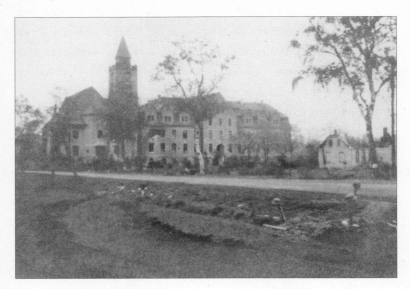

Our first location in Germany; British and German graves side by side in the foreground.

We crossed the pontoon bridge over the Rhine, the cost of which lay behind us marked with crosses, to our first destination beyond Rees. It did not come as a surprise when, a few days later, an order came asking us to return some of the things we had removed from Schloss Wissen. It was not couched in any vicious terms, but instead it sounded like a plea for our help and cooperation in this matter, however limited it might be. We were not surprised because we had seen the visitors' book at the schloss and among the pre-war guests were some very familiar English names. No doubt these had been used to persuade the military governorate to try and get some of her chattels returned. We thought the officers' mess should make the necessary and token sacrifice, and the kitchen stove and Persian carpet were therefore loaded on to a lorry to return across the Rhine and be dumped at the castle gates.

A few days later my unit was given leave. It seemed heaven-sent because I had begun to wonder how much longer it could go on without some short break from its daily ration of mangled flesh and bone and infinite sadness and tears.

I chose to go to Paris.

19

UNCOVERING A CONCENTRATION CAMP

APRIL–MAY 1945

On leave in Paris; return via Brussels to No. 3 CCS before rejoining No. 10 CCS near Bremen; VE-Day amid the horror of a concentration camp near Sandbostel; goodbye to No. 10 CCS and departure for Denmark

I hitched to Brussels and before anything else went to the public baths where I wallowed in deep hot water, soaping and soaping myself again and again. I could not remember when last I had had a bath, only that it was months before. Then I took the train to Paris where I arrived early in the morning. I hurried to Montmartre and rang the bell of Jeanne's flat. Ten days of happiness lay ahead, wandering in Paris and in the lush countryside of Marly-le-Roi, where the spring flowers were bright and the lilies of the valley nestled white in their green enclosing leaves. The tensions I lived with as a surgeon at war were easing, but I wondered whether they would ever leave me entirely. Now the backdrop to love was coloured red with the blood of gaping wounds and mutilated flesh.

Certain impressions were so vivid in my mind that they projected themselves in a non-stop performance from which, for the present, there was no escape.

I left Paris for Brussels on the night train. The carriages were packed with officers and men returning from leave, and though there were sleepers attached to the train these were reserved only for those on duty. It seemed certain to be a night in the corridor. There was no point in hastening to embark so I lingered on the platform and spoke to a South African officer who had just been discharged from hospital. He, too, was going back to Belgium, and a way to get there in comfort suddenly occurred to me. I found the controller of the sleeping cars and explained the predicament of this sick officer, for whom there was not even a seat on the train. I was the medical officer accompanying him and perhaps it would be possible to give us berths. Not much persuasion in French was needed for my story to be accepted and we were taken to a compartment which, in any case, had we not occupied it, would have remained unused. We stepped on to the platform at Brussels the following morning looking fresh and tidy instead of dishevelled and weary, like so many of our fellow travellers.

I had breakfast, went to the Blood Transfusion Service's base to ascertain the new location of my CCS, and drove to the airport where I hoped to find a plane going somewhere near. I was lucky. In about an hour a Dakota would be leaving for an airstrip very close to my unit. There were others going in the same direction and we climbed into the aircraft to make ourselves as comfortable as possible among the packing cases and stores with which the fuselage was filled. Over Germany, to the astonishment of all of us, and I think of the pilot and navigator too, we suddenly found ourselves in the midst of bursting ack-ack fire and the flames from the guns could be seen below. Some small isolated German battery was blasting a final protest, but happily its aim was bad.

For some reason the pilot was unable to land at the airstrip and was diverted miles away to another. Then he had to return to Brussels and it seemed easier for me to go back too. It was Saturday evening and I spent it happily with my friends at the Blood Transfusion Service who were delighted to see me back so soon.

There were no planes flying on the Sunday in my direction, so, as I was due back from leave that day, I hitchhiked by road. When we crossed into Germany this time, we were met by a different scene. Along the roads were groups of trudging people, quite happy, mostly men but women too. Some were civilians, or at least they were dressed in civilian clothes, but most were in the faded, tattered uniforms of many of the nations that had fought the Hun: French, Belgian, Russian, Polish, Greek and Norwegian too. Some were heading west and some east. A prisoner-of-war camp must have been liberated by the advancing armies and many of the prisoners had poured on to the roads.

It was dark when I finally arrived at No. 10 and the sky was filled with hundreds and hundreds of bombers on their way to pound Hamburg once again. In the distance the sky was soon aflame, as if the sun was setting in the east.

A wandering Russian known as Serge, large and formidable, had attached himself to the unit. He had been allowed to remain because each day he disappeared into the countryside and returned with sacks full of food. The previous day he had slit the throats of two geese and had donated them to the officers' mess, and they were roasting ready for the evening meal.

Two days later we were ordered to go to No. 3 CCS at Verden on the Weser, to which casualties from the battles in and around Bremen were being sent. We arrived and were told that we should not be needed until the evening, and that in the meantime, as there was no remaining room in the building in which the unit had been set up, I was to find billets in a house nearby. My attention was drawn to an order which stated that all German civilians must be evicted from any accommodation required by British troops.

We went in search of somewhere suitable but few houses remained undamaged. Eventually we found one, the only survivor in a small terrace. Officers in the RAMC had been issued with and ordered to carry revolvers in Germany. Most of the time mine and Bill's had been hidden under the back seat of our staff car, but on this occasion, just in case of any trouble, we had put them on our belts. My driver had a gun, too, and as I banged on the front door of the house I thought we would look very frightening to whoever answered our knock.

The door was opened by a woman in her thirties. Her startled and scared face as she looked at us showed we had produced the desired impression. In the very little German I knew I said, 'Wir kommen hier im hause in eine stunde. Alles ausgehen, alles in eine stunde.' Three small children had appeared to gather around their mother who burst into tears. She rushed back into the house and returned with an elderly lady who spoke near perfect English. I explained to her that we required her house and they would all have to leave.

'But where are we to go?' she asked. 'My daughter has three children and there are no houses left into which we can move. There's nowhere we can go. Both of us are widows. My daughter's husband was killed in Russia.'

'Let me see the house,' I said, and I inspected it. It had only a ground and a first floor, three rooms on each. I knew that, whatever the orders, I could not turn them out, and I knew, too, that not one of my unit would have wished me to do so. I spoke to the grandmother again. 'If you keep to the ground floor we will use the upper one and you won't have to leave. We will come back in about an hour so that you have time to move your things downstairs. We don't want any beds, we have our own.' She squeezed my hand, in tears.

It was very cold in the house and as there was a grate in one of the rooms upstairs we thought we would use it. 'Have you any coal?' I asked. 'Only a few lumps,' she replied. 'I will show you. We use a little oil for cooking.' She showed me her coal store, not more than a small half-scuttleful.

We took a set of keys and went in search of coal, deciding that somewhere there must be some. At the back of a derelict house we found a shed and through its shattered window we could see large piles of coal briquettes. The door was padlocked and we broke it down. We were loading some of the fuel on to the lorry when a man appeared; I did not like him. 'You cannot take that coal,' he said in broken English, 'eet is mine. You are stealing.' I reminded him what his nation had taken from many countries and that it was much more than sacks of coal. He persisted in his protest and again used the word stealing. I pulled out my revolver. 'Get out and stay out,' I said. 'We will now take every bit of your coal instead of the little we intended to remove.' He went and we loaded the lot. We took it back to our billet some distance away, carried enough for ourselves upstairs and restocked the coal shed below.

We had arrived at No. 3 CCS on 26 April and operated there till 2 May. Compared with past situations, casualties were very light and we had but five cases on the last day. I did not realise that the final soldier in this group was to be the last man wounded in battle upon who I was to operate. He was a prisoner of war with multiple wounds to his right leg and, sadly, his papers showed him to be a French national serving with the German army.

Now No. 10 CCS was east of the Weser not far from Bremen and we prepared to rejoin it. Before we vacated our billets we left some of our tinned rations on the table in our room because we knew that down below they were very short of food. How could we hate the old lady and her daughter and the three small children who smiled at us when we met?

The unit was not opened and everyone was wondering where the next move would take us. It was apparent from all the news bulletins that the end of the war in Europe was a matter of days, if not hours, away, and joining in the discussions we thought, very seriously, that we might soon be sailing for somewhere in the Far East.

May 6 14 Field Service Unit, 10 CCS, BLF

My dear Mum and Dad

And so it is, to all intents and purposes, over. At long last slaughter, murder, filth and dirt are nearing their end. No longer will our wards be filled with bodies rent and torn, with limbs shattered beyond repair. No longer will we want to weep at youth and its courage, and its lack of any word of reproach. No, throughout, all these months of this campaign, I have not heard one word of bitterness from any wounded man, when so much might have been said as pained and the thoughts of an unkind future caused such worry and anxiety.

But instead there has been a smile and an incredible lovely cheerfulness. Soon I suppose, I will be out of the army, but for all my grumbles, these years have not been entirely wasted, and I would not have wished to be anywhere else.

I have learnt much. Perhaps I am not the skilled surgeon that I might have been, but there are other matters that I have learned and benefited by. One I think is a great sympathy, and that I should never have learned at Kings. It has taken war in the field to teach me that.

The last letter that I wrote to you described a countryside practically untouched by war. This time I would describe such scenes of devastation by which standards any blitzed area in London looks built up.

I went to Bremen, a city the size of Bristol. The whole centre of the city is gutted. The rest lies a sprawling heap of ruins. I doubt whether there are 5 houses left out of 100 and these are scarred with broken windows and roofs. Frightened scared civilians scramble over the ruins. They have to me the appearance of rabbits scared by a pursuing dog. Oh yes, Germany is learning that war does not pay.

I am back with 10 CCS, but this afternoon I have to go to a concentration camp. I am not looking forward to it in the least. I have so many stories from people who have been there and seen so many photos that I would have preferred not to work in the centre of the lowest forms of human depravity. I know I shall want to vomit mentally and physically. 15,000 there are there – in conditions of filth, riddled with typhus and TB dying like flies. But there it is. I have to go, and now I must away to go and powder my clothes with anti-lice powder.

On 4 May a message came to the CO of the CCS, I believe from a field ambulance commander, requesting urgent assistance. A part of the division to which his unit was attached had discovered a concentration camp not far from a village called Sandbostel. My unit had a staff car and Bill and I were detailed to go and see what help was required and whether my unit would be adequate in providing the necessary aid. We passed through the village and were directed along a deserted road, little more than a lane, which passed through a heathland type of countryside. There were no farms or houses to be seen. Ahead was an enormous camp that looked, at first sight, like one for prisoners of war. It was surrounded by a very high double-barbed-wire fence, and along this, at intervals of some fifty yards or so, were observation towers with wrecked machine guns on the platforms. The camp gates were wide open. Inside were lines of long huts.

We were met and taken to one of these. Inside, the stench was almost insupportable. There were crude bunks on which emaciated figures clothed in striped pyjama-like uniforms were lying, several to each single space. They looked hardly human. A few were just able to prop themselves up on an elbow. The skin over their faces was drawn so tightly that any movement of their muscles made a hideous grimace. The hair on their heads was close cropped. Some held on to filthy scraps of black bread. On the floor lay dead bodies and those about to die, expressionless, hopeless, resigned. They lay in a scum of human excreta, liquid, slimy and stinking. A few still murmured and even moved a hand. Each hut was filled and overflowing. Outside were heaps of the old boots and shoes of those who had died. Not far away from the huts a large deep pit had been dug where bodies, little more than skin and bone, had been flung. They lay there in hundreds, their limbs sticking up in grotesque inhuman indignity.

A quarter of a mile from the camp was a true prisoner-of-war compound in which hundreds and hundreds of Russians were housed. They had been moved east as their armies had advanced from the west, but had been kept in reasonable condition. At the top of a small hill above the latter compound were rows of other huts which had been used by the guards and administrators of this complex of horror. There were some bunks in these, but hundreds of others could be quickly made and used as the basis of some form of hospital for those in the camp below.

The field ambulance, with its limited resources, had already done its very best. Already a marquee had been set up and some survivors had been rescued from the huts. There was other help. too, although it was, at least to start with, involuntary. A lorry had been sent to Bremen and any young woman seen on the streets was hustled into it and driven to the camp to aid in its clearance. There were to be many more lorry loads of these girls pressed into service. But the problem of caring for those who were still alive was going to be enormous, and most probably beyond the scope of a CCS. We rushed back. I think at first our CO scarcely believed what we had to tell, but he was soon convinced and the order for the CCS to move was given.

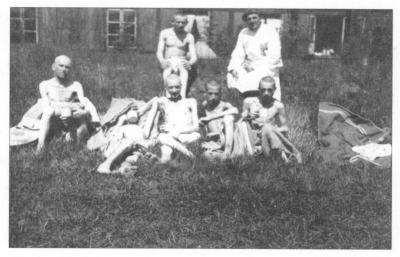

The author with Sandbostel survivors enjoying the sun.

At Sandbostel we worked from early morning till late at night, day after day, hard manual work with little doctoring about it. There was not a member of the unit, man or woman, who did not stretch themselves to the utmost. First, we had to build accommodation for hundreds in the huts on the hill. We hauled planks from wherever they could be found, sawed and nailed them to make bunks. In shifts we went down to the camp after powdering ourselves liberally with DDT. All working there were treated in this way to act as a protection against the lice.

In the huts we picked out those we thought stood a chance of life. The dying we had to ignore. They were all males in this concentration camp; those we chose were lifted on to stretchers and taken to ambulances which drove them to a large marquee a short distance away. Here their clothes were cut off to be burned and they were then lifted on to tables to be washed and shaved from head to toe by the women from Bremen. Spraying with DDT completed this initial cleansing, and on new stretchers they were taken to another ambulance for transport to the hospital, if so it could be called, on the hill. A blanket alone covered them, as there were no underclothes or pyjamas. In the wards sheets would be cut up to make loincloths. There we had no mattresses for them, only a blanket to ease the pressure from the hard boards. It took several days before the huts were all cleared, and during this time food and drink had to be provided for those left in their appalling state.

In the 'wards' conditions soon became hideous. Each room was large enough to accommodate about eight, but in some we had had to put as many as twenty-five. Most had diarrhoea and many typhus and tuberculosis. Those who could staggered from their bunks naked to answer every one of nature's calls on the floor. Those too weak or dying voided and evacuated in their bunks. It was a constant battle to keep some semblance of cleanliness and control but our nurses and orderlies never faltered in their efforts, and when we could every doctor helped them, too. There was infected spittle as well, everywhere. We could not continue like this and we begged our colonel to ask for a general hospital, with its large staff and tented accommodation, to be sent to help us. In the meantime more girls were brought from Bremen and German nurses joined us as well.

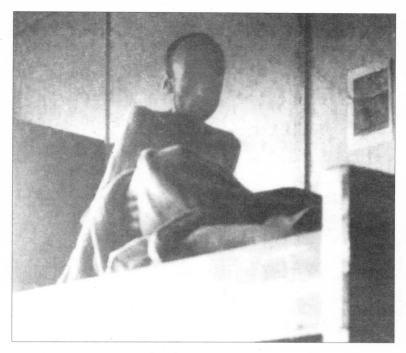

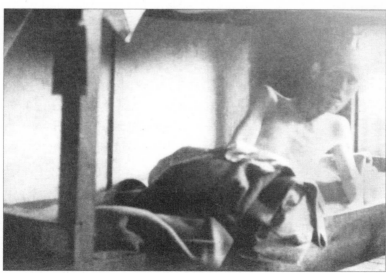

Survivors lay with little cover on hard wooden bunks.

Those in the camp were of all nationalities. There were French, Belgian and Dutch who had been partisans or had taken part in underground activities. There was even one Canadian who had been caught in France. But the majority were workers from Eastern European countries, who, after their usefulness had declined as the result of slow starvation and illness, had been sent to die in Sandbostel. They were of all ages, some hardly out of their childhood. There were doctors and other professional men too. More than a hundred of those we brought out of the camp died in the first week, but at the beginning there were others to put in their empty bunks.

There was little we could do medically. We were dealing with starvation, and the degradation of human dignity that only the months ahead would heal, and our endeavours now were to begin this return to normality. Months of unspeakable privation had reduced some to animal level. When a man lay dying, there were those in nearby bunks who would never take their eyes off him. They were waiting, ready to scramble across in order to seize his few possessions, often only scraps of bread, when they thought he was too near to death to cry out or to protect himself. We had tried to give the most emaciated intravenous drips of saline, plasma and even of blood. But these were usually torn down and drunk by others. If we gave medicine to one – and we had little enough – we had to give it to all. To start we prescribed it only to those who we thought might benefit, but the pathetic cries from so many who believed they were being overlooked made us give it to everyone.

Yet throughout this horror there were so many whose gentleness and patience inspired us. All their sufferings they bore with bravery and without complaint. Weak as they were they endeavoured to use bedpans, although so often failing, and to spit into scraps of paper. Dignity, decency and the behaviour of civilised society were no veneer to them. Such attributes lay deep and permanent and these had triumphed over every evil that had come to destroy them.

To add to our worries we had trouble with some of the Russian prisoners of war. Their camp, for which we were not responsible, was well separated from our own, but many persisted in wandering through our lines. Anything of use left outside any one of the wards disappeared. It was quite possible to prevent such losses, but it was the risk to the food being brought from the cookhouse to those wards that rapidly became an urgent problem. Our cooks were doing their utmost to prepare meals suitable for those who had starved for so long, only to have the containers seized as they carried them to the huts by groups of Russians. This plundering became so serious that an armed guard, with bayonet fixed, had to protect the containers as they were transferred to the wards.

★　★　★

VE-Day came and went. None of us had been in a frame of mind to give this wonderful occasion suitable celebration, and besides, we had no time. But as the days passed it began to seem that we too were gaining a victory. The number of those dying each day was falling. There were even traces of smiles on faces which for months and months had lost all power of expression. These men, and boys as well, started to sit up in their bunks and some even staggered outside to rest in the sun. Human dignity was returning and the animal life was being put away. Out of chaos slowly order was returning.

To my fellow officers and I it was now apparent that each victim required a thorough medical examination. There were many diseases, particularly tuberculosis, to be found among them and those suffering from this condition required urgent segregation. In the interests not only of themselves but also of all their fellow former prisoners, and of the nursing, medical and other staff caring for them, this had to be a priority. Among my own nursing orderlies one was to develop a severe lung infection, the undoubted result of working in this camp. However, we had neither the time, the personnel nor the facilities to carry out these examinations. There was no laboratory, no X-ray equipment. We were essentially a forward surgical unit and what we required was a general hospital.

In response to our many requests a fairly senior officer from the Corps Directorate of Medical Services came to see us. He was the first administrative medical officer we had seen and he was very clean. His batman must have spent a long time achieving that shine on the field boots below his breeches. We had not seen the like of such a uniform for many years and thought it had gone out with battledress. It was understandable that when he addressed us rather weary and slightly dirty lesser mortals that he should do it with some distaste. He had come to tell us the reasons why a hospital could not be sent to help us. His reception became stormy after this as we refuted all the arguments with which he had tried to support inaction. He walked out of the meeting saying he was not going to stay to be spoken to in this manner by junior officers, and we went back to our labours – furious.

8 May 14 Field Service Unit, 10 CCS, BLF Victory Day

Dear Mum and Dad,
Today with the end of all we've strived for I must write to you.

But we have little time to celebrate, and very little inclination for a party spirit as we are engaged in the biggest job we, as a CCS and attached units, have ever been asked to undertake. We are dealing with a horror concentration camp.

...

A representative of the army came up – a medical colonel, who had no wish to send a 1200 bed hospital and said he would not. We had the most stormy meeting and the colonel walked out of the conference. So I fulfilled my threat and went to the Corps Commander and told him all. This was no matter of pride. It was a matter of life and hope to hundreds, as well as the good health of all our unit.

The Corps Commander, a magnificent man, was charming. He saw the hospital for the second time, saw all the improvements and said he would get a 1200 bedder hospital, and would go to General Dempsey, the army commander.

So, my dears, I tell you this, because I know that you would like to see your son a Lt Col., but by such instances as this I am extremely unpopular with higher medical authority. But I have the support of every doctor here, as well as every other rank who somehow know the fight that I have had. And I will have done as good a job in argument as I have ever done in surgery, because many lives will be saved.

I must close now. Tonight I feel very calm, because I have worked hard in the last few days in a marvellous cause and I have fought bitterly now with process.

Our CCS is working marvellously – sisters to whom I take off my hat – everyone. This is a life and death struggle and we are winning. I'm glad as everyone here is that we can do our best for these poor lads – some only boys of sixteen – who have suffered years of the terror and horror of hell.

A few days later the Corps Commander, Lieutenant-General Sir Brian Horrocks, came to visit us. His name was legendary in the Corps and there must have been few, if any, men who would not have followed him to the death. Tall and handsome, he had the reputation of being a brilliant tactician, and one who exercised every possible consideration to the officers and men under him. Respect and admiration he did not command: it came naturally and willingly from all.

We talked to him about our problems, showed him our wards and our patients. Turning to the very senior Army Medical Service officer who had accompanied him he said, 'I think these chaps need a hospital. We'll arrange that when we get back.' We had won our plea.

The general had fought and been a prisoner himself in Russia after the First World War, and he spoke the language fluently. He had been told of the problems we were having with the Russian prisoners of war and they were assembled so that he could talk to them. His words were greeted with merry laughter, approval and hand-clapping, and from that time on we had no further trouble and the food containers went to the wards unguarded and were not attacked.

In my unit's lorries, tentage and equipment for a twelve-bedded ward had not, as yet, been unloaded, and towards the end of May I decided that it should be used. To remove even this small number of patients from the primitive bunks and surroundings in the huts, or wards as they had become, seemed better than nothing, but to select the few who would be transferred was difficult. Eventually, with the help of our sister, a list was made. It included our youngest patient, a Hungarian, about fifteen years old.

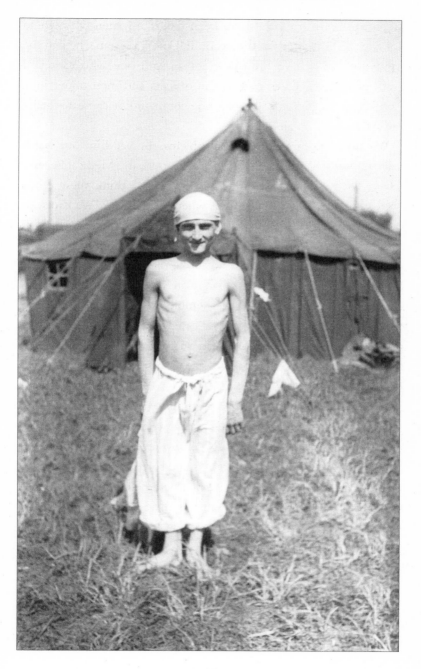

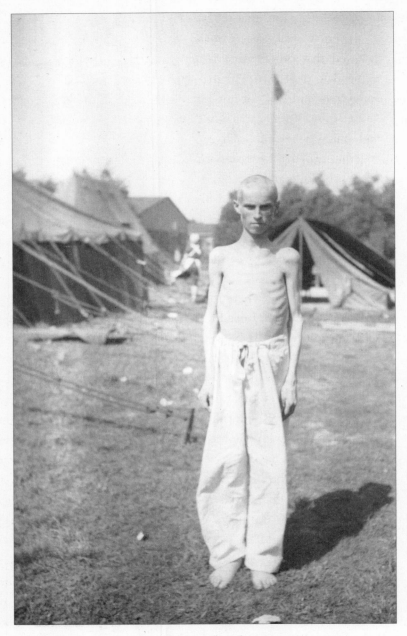

Two of the youngest survivors of the Sandbostel concentration camp.

We were anxious that the marquee should not be very obvious as we knew well what would happen if certain of our patients believed that others were being given comforts and treatment better than their own. The marquee was therefore pitched behind some trees and was not noticeable from the huts. Into it the beds and mattresses were carried to be made up with clean white sheets and pillowcases, and each was covered with red blankets. My orderlies searched for boxes and packing cases and one was placed at each bedside and covered with lint from our store. Then they went into the fields around the camp to pick wild flowers and a bunch of these in a jar was placed on every table. A glass of water, a few biscuits and a pair of pyjamas to each bed completed our arrangements and the ward looked quite lovely. We were ready to start the transfer.

I went to the hut where I knew the boy was and beckoned him from the door. He at once looked scared as if wondering whether some further horror lay ahead. Outside the door I took his hand. He spoke a little English. 'Don't worry,' I said, 'just come with me.' I led him to the marquee and he stopped, astonished. I took him to one of the beds and said, 'This is for you.' He fingered the sheets, touched the flowers, flung his arms around me and then fell on the bed sobbing with emotion. My eyes were full of tears, too, and I wondered how anyone could have treated this boy so cruelly. I went outside to be alone for a little while, and then, one by one, we brought the others over. As they all settled into their beds with smiles of delight I do not think there could have been a happier ward in all the world.

The hospital that was to take over from us started to arrive. I was told that my unit would soon be sent to Denmark, but I was to take only one lorry and, instead of the staff car, a Jeep, which I was to collect. We were to hand in all our theatre equipment and to take only the small tents necessary for our own use.

A very long association with No. 10 CCS was nearing its end. I had commanded it for many weeks in the desert, knew all its personnel so well, and had admired them for all they had done, not least in this concentration camp. We had a team of superb nurses, led by an Australian, Nancy Kinsella. She had been in England at the outbreak of war and had immediately joined the Army Nursing Service and been sent to No. 6 General Hospital in France. It was her personality and her dedication to the wounded that had done so much to help this CCS perform with distinction, from Bayeux to Sandbostel.

Somehow, certain of our patients learned of the imminent departure of myself and my unit, and a Frenchman asked me whether he and his countrymen could meet us. Of course I said yes. The next day they lined up in the ill-fitting pyjamas which had now been provided. They were very thin but they were on the road to recovery. Their leader made his speech of thanks for what we had done. 'We will never forget,' he said – and they did not, because later I was to receive the Croix d'Honneur for my work among them.

Could the whole German nation be as depraved as those who had produced this hell on earth? From the little I had seen of the civilian population I could not believe this. When the girls who had been swept off the streets of Bremen and brought to Sandbostel – there were more than two hundred of them – were told, after working there for over two weeks, that they could return home should they wish, only a handful accepted the offer. Perhaps these few had very pressing reasons, but the others said they would remain until they were no longer required. There was hope for Germany.

We were given a wonderful farewell dinner and on 28 May we were on our way to Denmark with a week in which to make the journey. With the exception of one day, when I had had the privilege of being asked to see our Corps commander who was suffering from the flare-up of a terrible wound he had received in Tripoli, I had not left the camp since we first arrived. Now we were going down the lane to the main road and I was driving the new Jeep. Smoke and flames were billowing from the huts of the concentration camp as, finally, the evidence of its evil was being destroyed with fire.

20

CLEARING THE WOUNDED IN DENMARK

JUNE–JULY 1945

To Copenhagen via Cuxhaven; assessing the German
wounded in Zealand hospitals; usefulness of cigarettes; goodbye
to No. 14 FSU and to Hanover via Flensburg

Seven days lay ahead before we were due to report at Copenhagen,
and it had been suggested to us that before we left Sandbostel we
spend a part of that time in Cuxhaven. Here, apparently, full facilities
were available for officers and men on leave. So we took the road
through Bremen, a city I had visited before the war. I remembered
its beautiful seventeenth-century houses, carved and decorated at
the time it was a member of the Hanseatic League of trading ports.
Fortunately it was only the dock area which had been devastated;
most of the Alte Stadt survived and the damage could be repaired.

We had entered Germany only a few months before and
back then the sight of Cleves and Goch was, as my corporal had
remarked, 'Just the job.' But the war was now over. Such feelings

had evanesced as quickly as the smell of smoke and cordite from a gun that had fired its last shell. Now there was a sense of uplifting relief at the sight of any old building, created by the skill, pride and craftsmanship of centuries ago, which had survived, and which still stood, inspiring and beautiful.

We arrived in Cuxhaven to find that no leave centre existed, but a field ambulance offered us its warm hospitality although they were moving on the following day. Clubs, however, had been opened, one for other ranks and one for the officers, the latter in the Yacht Club. That night Bill and I sat down to dinner in the dining room there. We were served by Germans soup, an enormous helping of halibut, apple tart and plentiful Rhenish wine. Not many months ago, I mused, these same servants, most elderly, must have been serving the same menu to their own officers who had just come off their U-boats or who were preparing for another mission against the Allied convoys in the Atlantic. Had they had their way they would have been dining in the Royal Yacht Squadron at Cowes and the swastika would have been flying at the masthead.

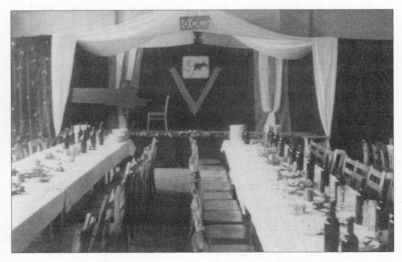

Victory party, Cuxhaven.

29 May 14 FSU attached 32 CCS BLA

Dear Mum and Dad,

How rapidly has the face of the world changed in these last few weeks. What seemed well nigh impossible a year ago, lapses back into the ordinary, unmarvelled and unwondered at. I wonder how many of us thought 5 years ago that victory would come as completely as it has.

When we leave here we go up into Denmark. There is no doubt about the slogan "Join the army and see the world". This is certainly a spot of luck for us, for except on duty visiting this country is strictly forbidden. But in addition to just seeing it it will be grand to get away from the artificial atmosphere of Germany. The army is confronted with a very great problem in its policy of non-fraternisation, or fratting as it is called, right though it probably is. But if thousands of troops are dumped down in a country with no fighting to do, then as sure as the dawn follows the night, the boys and girls will get together... I suppose that officially we must regard all Germans as fundamentally bad. But at the hospital at Sanbostel for example where there are some 150 German nurses and 25 young girls who have worked , there is no doubt about it, exceptionally well, it is difficult to believe that all are bad. And 10 CCS whose personnel are a gullible lot, certainly don't think so.

We left the port and on the road to Hamburg passed an enormous prisoner-of-war camp that must have held thousands. Through its gates long columns of defeated German soldiers still straggled, some on horseback and some, unable to endure the march, crowded into old horse-drawn farm carts, There was no goose step now, no steel-helmeted Nazi arrogance, no pride in their march, only sullen impassiveness as they went to captivity. No other army transport was on the road and we saw no British guards. We hoped too there was no Nazi fanatic lurking in the camp who wished to reopen the war with a shot at us as we drove by.

Hamburg was almost a ghost city with street upon street of stark ruins, which once were houses and shops and public buildings. Slabs of masonry were the only tombstones for bodies still lying beneath the debris. Here and there a front room had been shored up to form a shop where a few basic foods were being sold. It was an awesome and depressing sight and we were glad to leave.

Beyond Flensburg we crossed into a country with tidy farms and neat towns, unspoiled by the war's devastation. Only periodic columns of German troops marching south to the frontier told of the grim years of occupation suffered by the Danes. They had not been short of food and their towns remained intact, but for five years they had had to live under the domination of the Nazis. From those to whom we spoke we learned of their hatred and of their one desire to see them all out of the country as quickly as possible. It was to help in this evacuation that we were being sent to Copenhagen.

For two days we camped just below the bridge linking Funen to the mainland, bathing, reading, sleeping and recovering from our work at Sandbostel. We went on, feeling cleansed by the cold water of the western end of the Baltic Sea.

A ferry linked Funen to Zealand, the largest of the islands that make up Denmark, and boarding this with passes with which we had been provided for our two vehicles and ourselves, we made our way to the promenade deck. The windows of the ship's dining room faced on to this and we could see the stewards carrying large dishes of *smorrebrod*, roast chicken, ham and gateaux to the tables.

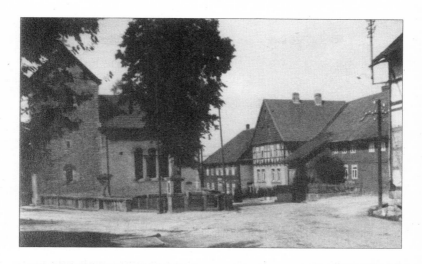

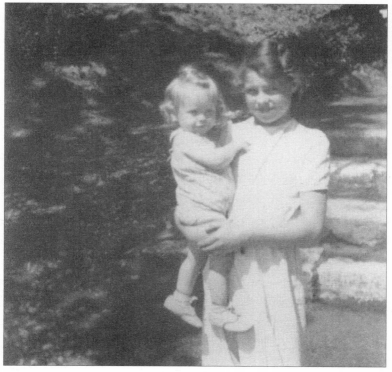

Dankelheim village, near the border with Denmark.

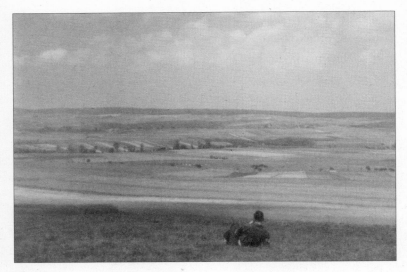

The author at large, enjoying the scenery.

Our eyes must have been protruding and certainly our mouths were watering, but we had no money. It did not take me long to decide that we would all go to lunch and sort out the matter of the bill when it arrived. When the bill was duly delivered at the end of a wonderful meal, I told the waiter that I had no money but would sign the bill and forward the cost as soon as I reached Copenhagen.

'Have you any cigarettes?' he asked.

'Yes,' I replied. 'But why?'

'You can pay with those at the rate of ten kroner for twenty,' he answered. We were astounded at this but rapidly counted out the necessary number. When we were back on deck congratulating ourselves on such good fortune, a diminutive soldier, whom I had noticed in the dining room, came up to me, saluted, and in a marked Scottish accent said, 'Canna I have a wee word with you, sir?' I went with him a few yards away from the rest of my unit. 'I saw you paying for that meal with cigarettes,' the soldier said. I suddenly thought that I must have contravened some army regulation concerning cigarettes with which I was not familiar, and that I was going to be reported for the offence. He went on, 'You're new to Denmark, sir, but I've been here for a wee while now. The rate of exchange is one kroner per cigarette and that waiter cheated you. He only gave you half a kroner. I thought I ought to let you know the correct rate. There's nothing you can't buy with cigarettes in Denmark.' I thanked him profusely, we exchanged salutes and I hurried to tell my unit the good news.

We arrived in Copenhagen and reported to the medical office there. Accommodation was allocated to us, and Bill and I were to go to the Hotel Kongen af Danmark. We were to report on the following morning to be briefed by the colonel about our duties.

That evening, in the most comfortable of hotels, we sent letters to all our friends in England, and those of our relatives who we thought might respond, telling them of our complete lack of cigarettes and asking them whether they would mind sending the odd thousand or so. But until the golden currency started to arrive, unhappily we would have to visit the Army Pay Office the following day.

We met the colonel and he told us what our duties would involve. We had to visit every German hospital in Zealand (and there were many) in order to assign every wounded man to one of four categories: those who could not be moved; those who could be sent to Germany by ambulance train; those who could be evacuated by lorry; and those who were able to walk. He said that the Danish government were exercising pressure to rid Denmark of all Germans at the earliest possible time, so the sooner we finished our assessment the better.

We left to visit the first hospital accompanied by an interpreter. Both of us felt that our reception by the colonel had not been as warm as it might have been. He wore breeches and field boots and carried no campaign ribbon, only that of the jubilee medal. Perhaps he was a friend of the last newly arrived colonel from England with whom we had exchanged heated words at Sandbostel and he had been informed of that episode.

Our task was going to be formidable if we were to do it fairly and efficiently, which was our intention. It would involve seeing, if not examining, thousands of soldiers in order to decide into which category each should be placed. To start we would deal with those hospitals actually in Copenhagen and later visit those in the outlying regions of the island. Sometimes it would take several days to complete the list in a large hospital, whereas in the smaller units our inspection would require only one visit.

From each commanding officer we obtained the names of his wounded men and then proceeded to our inspection. Compared with our own wounded in base hospitals, the condition of these Germans, some of whom had come from the Eastern and others from the Western fronts, was deplorable. They were ill nursed, their wounds covered only with paper dressings soaked through with discharges, and every amputation we saw was of a guillotine type, in which the skin, the muscles and the bones had all been transected at the same level. This was the technique of amputation at the time of Trafalgar and Waterloo, and it left a raw area over which the skin would finally grow only after many months. It was a method rightly forbidden in the British Army; instead we fashioned flaps of skin, which would cover the exposed region left on completion of the amputation.

We worked steadily, but not hurriedly, through each ward making our lists. On our decision the future of any of these severely wounded soldiers might rest. When we felt uncertainty as to the category into which a man should fall, as we did in many cases, we always gave him the benefit of the doubt so that his transfer to Germany, if he could be moved, would be made as comfortable as possible. Each evening we handed in our lists to the office and the following day the evacuation of the hospital concerned would commence.

The hospitality extended to us by our Danish hosts was abounding. Each night we were pressed with invitations, but the experience of a few made us, for self-preservation's sake, decline many. The Danes were at long last free from the tyranny of occupation and their celebrations had not yet ceased. These often commenced in the early-evening hours and continued till dawn. Husbands became parted from wives and wives from husbands and an unmarried officer was in as much demand as water in a desert. Agreeing to be a guest at a party was as dangerous as canoeing through the rapids of a river in spate and required great skill to navigate it safely. One did not wish to hazard that safety too often.

Copenhagen was a lovely city in which to stroll and window-shop or idle in the Tivoli or along the waterfront where the mermaid sat. There seemed to be no poverty, even in the dock areas. Every 'working man's' house or flat was 'middle class' and there was an abundance of food. Only the person too idle to pick up a golden coin from the pavement could be poor there. The social services appeared to be in advance of our own and the civilian hospitals we visited were new by comparison with so many of the old buildings in England. We wondered whether the Danes had founded a modern Utopia. Yet it seemed a country without a challenge to its people. They had no mountains to climb, no rivers to navigate or forests to explore, and few minerals or fuels to extract from the earth. Perhaps it was Denmark's lack of these exacting features that made life in Paris seem almost puritanical compared with the hedonism of this city.

Most of the German doctors we met and who accompanied us during our inspection of the wounded were courteous and helpful, but there were a few who were churlish and we knew that their loyalty to Nazism had not been diminished in defeat. We had completed our work in some two-thirds of the hospitals when we encountered one in which this attitude was predominant, and through our interpreter we complained to the senior medical officer of the lack of cooperation from his juniors. Nevertheless, we carefully prepared our list and handed it into the office in Copenhagen.

As we reported to our colonel on the following morning to receive our instructions for the day's work ahead, we were surprised to see some of the same officers about whom we had complained emerging from his office. He told us that the German doctors had disagreed with the categories into which we had placed some of their wounded, that he had accepted their objections and had accordingly amended the list we had submitted. We could scarcely believe what he was saying. It was true that every medical officer had the right, indeed the duty, to obtain the best possible conditions for the wounded for whom he was responsible, but for our colonel to accept their opinion without giving us any opportunity to defend our own was preposterous. We protested very strongly, but the alterations to the list remained and we left the office in some heat.

If that was the way in which our carefully made decisions were to be discarded there was no longer any point in making them. In future we would call on the commanding officer of the hospital we were visiting and instruct him to draw up the necessary list; we would collect it in the evening and would occupy the intervening hours in other ways. Apart from exploring the rest of the island and bathing, we had business to attend to: the cartons of cigarettes were starting to arrive and negotiations for their exchange had to be organised. We never entered the wards of a German hospital again.

15 June 14 FSU c/o ADM/S Shaef Military Mission, Copenhagen, Denmark

Dear Mum and Dad,

I have sent home 90 eggs, and I hope by the time you get this letter they will have arrived. There is no difficulty at all about sending them. The only difficulty is the cartons which are in short supply. So if you could let me have them back as soon as possible so much the better. I hope to be able to get some cheese off soon...

I cannot pretend that this job is very difficult. In fact not only does it not require two doctors to do it, it doesn't require any at all, and any good sergeant could do it with the greatest of ease...

No wonder they say 'we're short of doctors, and we can't demobilise you'. It makes me very angry, but as the food and drink is good, and the atmosphere is pleasant, we refrain from criticism for fear of being sent back to Germany. This is what it consists of. I and Bill – we don't both need to go but with two it's more fun – go to a German hospital. We see the chief German doctor, we say 'How many patients have you here fit to move to Germany? Let me have a list of names. Tomorrow we will take them on the first stage of the journey.' We then take a token look at the hospital, retire to the local pub for a pint while they are preparing the list, then we collect it, and off to Copenhagen. Now if an office boy couldn't do that? Can you credit it? ... But if someone is going to do a soft job – it's this little boy this time! ...

Lucienne [the Parisian actress my father met in 1940 whom he had now married] is making the first steps for home. I think it will take some time but probably she will be home before myself. I know that when you meet her you will be very very fond of her, and I look forward so much to her meeting my old Derby and Joan. It will be a happy day.

My love to you both.

There could have been only a few, if any, soldiers, who had not written home as I had to ask for cigarettes to be sent. The Army Post Office was deluged with parcels. It must have come as a great surprise to many relatives of confirmed non-smokers to learn that their dear ones had resorted to the weed. I saw a very senior officer who had a rather bad abscess. He also had a cough and I asked him whether he smoked much. 'I've never smoked,' he replied, but there on his table, only partially concealed by papers, were several cartons of Churchman's No. 1, and these rather superior cigarettes commanded a higher price than the ordinary Player's or Wills.

The Danes had been without cigarettes for years and it would have been reasonable to suppose that their desire to smoke had long passed. But this was not so and they continued to crave. It was impossible to walk down any street without being asked whether we had any to sell. My post was abundant and I was able to purchase a fox-fur jacket for Jeanne and a tea service for a friend in England who was getting married. Our colleagues in the RAF were always willing to take our parcels home.

I had hoped to find a cine camera but this was not easy. The Germans had seen to that. Eventually I was offered one for twelve hundred cigarettes and I bought it. When I examined it more closely back at the hotel I found that its spring motor only worked for some fifteen seconds on each wind, and on the frame I noticed the words 'Sûreté Générale'. At some time the camera had belonged to the French police and had been used to take short shots, presumably at the scene of some crime. It was no good for my purposes. My first call the following morning was to the Dane from whom I had purchased the camera. I explained its limitations, pointed out that it was quite useless for ordinary work and asked whether he would return the cigarettes. He said that he could not do this as he had disposed of them. 'But,' he said, 'I could give you a box of fully fashioned rayon stockings instead.' I had heard how difficult it was to buy anything like this in England, and thinking that these were better than a useless camera, I took them.

That evening I was with some RAF friends and I was telling them about this incident.

'Do you want to get rid of them?' one asked.

'Well yes, I do,' I replied.

'All right, I'll take them. They are just what our chaps want. They'll sell at a packet of twenty a pair and I'll take ten per cent.'

The deal was clinched and the following day all were duly disposed of and most of my capital remained intact.

I had told my parents that I was in Copenhagen and to my astonishment received a reply from them informing me they had heard that my brother was there too. I managed to find him and we greeted each other for the first time since before the outbreak of war. We dined together and talked far into the night, catching up in those few hours on the events of several years. He had first served in minesweepers, then undergone training as a gunnery officer before transferring to a corvette. This meant that month after month, rarely free of seasickness, in a small, lurching and plunging ship, always wet, night and day, and never out of his clothes, he and his crew had waited for the explosion of a torpedo which would blow their ship out of the water It never came, but it came to others of the escort and to many of the merchant vessels they convoyed.

He had been transferred to the SS *Queen Elizabeth* as chief gunnery officer. It seemed strange that a solicitor in his mid-thirties should have been in charge of the defence of the largest and most expensive passenger ship ever to have been launched. Later he joined the *Viceroy of India*, which, towards the end of 1942, was to transport troops to North Africa. These were landed safely, but on the homeward run the ship was torpedoed. Damaged and disabled but still afloat, it became a sitting target for German bombers and it was hit and sunk. It was during this engagement that Arthur received his severe head wound. I asked him whether the dive-bombers had been fitted with the air brakes we had watched being developed behind the tea-house on the road between Ware and Cambridge. He smiled. 'I really didn't have time to see.'

By the end of June all the German hospitals on Zealand had been visited and I received a posting to No. 29 General Hospital in Hanover, where I was to be the officer in charge of the surgical division. From the date of the order, I was promoted, so had to buy two stars and sew them on my epaulettes above my crowns. Bill, who was some years older than I, was to return to England; the rest of my unit, who had been attached to a CCS while we were visiting the hospitals, were for the time being to remain there.

No. 14 FSU had come to the end of its service and on the eve of my departure we all dined together. I felt very proud of these young men with whom I had worked so closely. They had done a very difficult, unfamiliar and often harrowing job, and the unit's success, efficiency and high repute had been dependent as much on them as it had its two officers. I had recommended Corporal MacGregor to be mentioned in dispatches and Lance-Corporal Jones for the British Empire Medal, and both recommendations had been approved. We talked of the past and of the future until it was very late, and the next morning I loaded my gear into the Jeep and started my drive back to Germany.

Over the border I stopped for a short time in Flensburg, a small town lying at the head of a long deep fjord. It was the most northerly of all German ports and now its harbour was filled with merchant and naval ships anchored in surrender. The town with its old gabled houses and narrow streets had been little damaged.

Here in the last few days of the war, Karl Doenitz, at one time the ill-famed commanding admiral of Germany's U-boats and Hitler's unquestioning stooge, had set up that country's final government after being nominated successor by the Führer immediately before his suicide. From this port Himmler, following his dismissal by Doenitz, had escaped in disguise, with patched eye and shaven upper lip, only to be arrested beyond Hamburg and to kill himself by crushing the vial of cyanide he had secreted in his mouth. This, too, was the town from which the admiral had telegraphed final instructions to Jodl in Reims, authorising him to sign the deed of the unconditional surrender of all forces on that Monday morning of 7 May. There would always be history here as, since 1918, there had been at Compiègne in France. I wanted to remember it.

EPILOGUE

JULY–OCTOBER 1945

Final posting to a hospital in Hanover; return to England; discharge at
Albany Street Barracks; back on the wards at King's College Hospital

I arrived at my new hospital in Hanover. It was housed in a cold
dreary building in the suburbs of the wrecked city. The mess was
comfortless and its amenities seemed modelled to match the austerity
in which, at that time, the Germans were living. I did not think that a
combatant unit would have tolerated it and I soon saw that this was
so when the medical staff of our hospital, including, of course, our
sisters, were invited to a dance given by a Scottish regiment a few
miles away. They, quite rightly, were living very comfortably. Their
commanding officer had seen to that but ours seemed to have no
interest in material comfort. From my point of view it did not really
matter as I knew that my release, based on age and years of service,
was not far off, but I felt sorry for those who had to stay. I did my
best to improve matters but without much success.

There was little work to do in the hospital. We were dealing with a fit young garrison and it was only the occasional accident or an acute abdominal condition, such as appendicitis, which required attention in the operating theatre. I could hardly wait to return to civilian hospital practice.

6 July Major S Aylett 14 FSU c/o ADM/S. Shaef Military Mission, Copenhagen, Denmark

My dear John [Gilpin],
I wish to god I could see an end of my army career. I have never had one regret during actual war time, but this frigging about here is just scandalous.

Thank you for the cigarettes which arrived safely and of course your letter too. If you could manage another 500 I'd be very grateful. They are like gold here.

Now firstly I have a great piece of news. I hope that by now my everloving will be in England. With her customary complete control of the situation she seems to have fixed all her affairs in Paris, shut her flat, sold the furniture, and decided that Stanley or no Stanley, she'd better get to London. So as soon as you possibly can you go and visit her because there is none of my very great pals whom I would like better to welcome her...

I do not know when I shall get out of this army. I hope soon because although this visit to Denmark is all very pleasant, I want to get back to civilian surgery. I understand that King's are asking for me back which I am very happy to know. Perhaps in spite of a few blacks to my name I may yet get on the staff. That, I need hardly say, would be the greatest honour that could come my way, because I am very fond of King's...

I have not heard from Mac for some time, but I do not think that I shall be surprised to see an alliance with Dorothy. But what a sorry plight this war has made of so many marriages. John, we must hang on to what is golden, cherish it, and never ever take is as a matter of course. People as well as things, that are lovely and beautiful must be looked after, so that beauty and loveliness doesn't fade in the drab ticking away of time.

Do write again soon and you'll have a happy visit to my everloving

Ever yours,

Stanley

I was sent to Paris for several days to attend an Allied conference on gunshot wounds of the abdomen and to recount my experiences and views on how best they should be treated. There I stayed in luxury at the Hotel Vendôme, which, with the British Officers' Club beside the Embassy, where champagne cocktails could be drunk, compensated for our Hanoverian mess for a few days.

In October the day of my return to England arrived. I travelled to Ostend by way of Cologne. A few years before the war I had taken part in a hockey festival there, and in those ten days I had come to know the city fairly well. I remembered its old houses and streets and its lovely thirteenth-century town hall, but now all were rubble and all that remained from the past was the cathedral with its twin towers rising high into the sky.

At Ostend the shops, brightly lit, were open late into the evening and filled with all sorts of things to buy, and with our purchases some fellow officers and I sailed next morning for Dover. The customs men were there to meet us. I had bought a pair of binoculars in Copenhagen, admittedly with cigarettes, but I had to pay five pounds duty on them, a considerable sum in those days. I did not tell the officer of the Walther pistol I had in my pocket. I had taken this from the body of a Belgian soldier who had died of his wounds in the little boat in which we had put to sea from near Dunkirk in 1940 and had carried it with me for the rest of the war. The only shots I had ever fired from it were those I used to destroy a mad dog in Alexandria. Later, and very reluctantly, I surrendered the weapon to the police.

We arrived in London and were taken to Albany Street Barracks where we were given food and clothing coupons and discharge papers. From there, my final and short journey in an army-transport truck took me to Olympia to choose a civilian outfit. My selections were packed in a cardboard box and my service with the army had finished.

I went outside to be accosted by a number of touts wishing to give me eleven pounds for the clothing. It was of pretty inferior quality and I doubted whether I should ever use it, but I would rather have thrown it away than sell it to these spivs, for whom, I supposed, the war had been one long profitable black market. I told them to be off in vernacular terms, hailed a taxi and drove home.

A week later, just six years and two months from the day I had left my teaching hospital, King's College, I was happily back at work there.

Army Form X212

RELEASE CERTIFICATE
EMERGENCY COMMISSIONED OFFICERS—REGULAR ARMY
(CLASS " A " RELEASE IN U.K.)

(1) A/Lt.Col. S. O. AYLETT (104033)

R. A. M. C.

The above-named has been granted (2) 113 days' leave commencing 13.10.45 and is, with effect from 3.2.46 released from military duty under Regulations for Release from the Army, 1945.

Uniform may be worn during leave, except in Eire, but will not be worn after leave has expired, except as may be specially authorised.

As an officer holding an Emergency Commission in the Regular Army he will be placed on the Unemployed List from the effective date of release, with liability to recall to military duty until the end of the present emergency.

During the continuance of the emergency officers will notify in writing any change of permanent address to the Under Secretary of State, The War Office, to whom applications for permission to leave the United Kingdom will also be made.

The War Office   By Command of the Army Council,
A.M.D.I.

3 0 NOV 1945

Initials ....

IF FOUND. Please enclose this certificate in an unstamped envelope and address it to the Under Secretary of State, The War Office, London, S.W.1.

NOTICE. This document is Government property. Any person being in possession of it without authority or excuse is liable under Section 156(9) of the Army Act to a fine of £20 (twenty pounds), or imprisonment for six months, or to both fine and imprisonment.

8313

Major (Acting Lieutenant-Colonel) S. O. Aylett was released from the army on 13 October 1945.

I feel I cannot let you leave 21 Army Group on your return to civil life without a message of thanks and farewell. Together we have carried through one of the most successful campaigns in history, and it has been our good fortune to be members of this great team. God Bless you and God speed.

B. L. Montgomery

BLA · 1945

FIELD MARSHAL
COMMANDER IN CHIEF

A thank you from Field Marshal Montgomery,
Commander-in-Chief,
Twenty-First Army Group

10, Upper Wimpole Street, W.1,

2nd Sept., 1946.

LT.-COL. S. O. AYLETT, R.A.M.C.

I have had the pleasure of knowing Lt.-Col. Aylett for almost six years. In the early stages of the war I heard many good things of his work both in B.E.F. and in M.E.F., and was therefore delighted to find that he was to be one of my surgeons in 21st Army Group.

During the campaign in N.W. Europe, from early days in Normandy to the occupation stage in Germany, I had many opportunities of seeing him and his work. Until the end of hostilities he was C.O. of a Field Surgical Unit, and in view of his previous very considerable experience of war surgery, was constantly in the thick of the battle and got through an enormous amount of very good work. There was a natural tendency for the worst and most difficult cases to be sent to the more experienced war surgeons, and to my personal knowledge Lt.-Col. Aylett has tackled more than his share of these with what to him must be most gratifying results.

He has a very sound clinical sense and good judgment, is quite imperturbable in an emergency, his surgical technique is most sound and meticulous—being founded on an exceptionally good anatomical basis, his after-care of his patients was particularly praiseworthy.

As C.O. of his Unit he showed a definite flair for simple efficient organisation and administration and was deservedly popular with his fellow-officers, his men and his patients alike.

With a mind of his own, an equable temperament and a sense of humour, I found him a most loyal and invaluable colleague. I am sure both as a man and a surgeon he would be a distinct acquisition to any hospital staff. I have no hesitation in thoroughly recommending him.

(Signed) A. E. PORRITT,

C.B.E., M.Ch., F.R.C.S.

Surgeon to Out-Patients and Assistant Director,
Surgical Unit, St. Mary's Hospital.

Surgeon to His Majesty,
late Consulting Surgeon 21st Army Group.

Letter of reference, 2 September 1946, from A. E. Porritt, who had known the author during the war.

AFTERWORD

My father left the army with the rank of lieutenant-colonel. It was a commission he had been offered before with the direction of a military hospital, but he had never wanted to be a 'base wallah', preferring to work alongside those on the front line. It was for these services with his Field Surgical Unit in Europe that he was appointed MBE, and in 1952 the Franco-British Friendship Society awarded him the Croix d'Honneur for his work at Sandbostel concentration camp.

He returned for a brief period to King's College Hospital, where he had qualified, but he eventually had to look elsewhere to advance his career, something he regretted. With the start of the National Health Service, he was appointed consultant surgeon to the Gordon Hospital, a branch of Westminster Hospital. He remained here until his retirement, though he also worked and taught as a consultant surgeon at the Metropolitan and Potter's Bar Hospitals and at the Manor House Trade Union Hospital in Golders Green.

As a surgeon he was known to have the fastest fingers in the business and he developed a special interest in the treatment of colitis, a severe inflammatory disease of the bowel. Conventional practice at the time was to remove the diseased intestine, leaving patients with the humiliation and difficulty of managing an ileostomy, an exterior waste bag. My father pioneered a treatment to avoid this but when he published his results in 1966 they were challenged by the medical establishment, which believed that patients would develop intractable diarrhoea and risk cancer in the retained bowel. The attack became personal, not least, he told me, because, for the private sector, there were financial as well as medical issues at stake. I remember him gleefully reading out one of the letters published in the *British Medical Journal* in which the writer suggested it was perhaps time for him to retire. He carried on, the patients kept coming, and his procedure, ileo-rectal enastomosis, has now become standard, something which earned him international renown.

He travelled widely among the community of surgeons, visiting America and the Soviet Union and regularly returning to France. In 1952 he became an Honorary Member of the American Society of Colon and Rectal Surgeons, and in 1961 he was recognised by the American Proctologic Society for an 'outstanding contribution' to the field. In 1974 he was made an honorary member of the French Academy of Surgeons, which because of the affinity he felt with France, was an honour he particularly treasured. At home he held office as President of the Section for Coloproctology at the Royal Society of Medicine, and President of the Chelsea Clinical Society.

Many times, my father's reputation has caught up with me. While supporting my Kurdish friend who had terminal breast cancer, her consultant at Hammersmith Hospital asked if I was related to the consultant, Stanley Aylett. He then turned to her: 'Your friend's father was one of those rare men who dedicated his life and immense skills to make people like you better. And that is how we will care for you here.' Eight years after his death, whilst undergoing tests at the Whittington Hospital, the consultant asked if I was related. I told him that I was his daughter. 'How extraordinary,' he said. 'I'm now treating one of his patients, an elderly man in his nineties.'

These encounters have strengthened my sense of being linked in a human chain, and while working on this book I finally decided to visit Sandbostel. Since I first knew of it, the name had stayed inside me with all the long shadows cast by its associations, yet through all the years I had never tried to locate it. The village lies between Bremen and Hamburg, and the camp is just outside, discreetly signposted, Lager Sandbostel, Stalag XB. Later I learnt how the local community had not wanted to accept the existence of the 'horror' camp, though the existence of a prisoner-of-war camp and the thousands who had died here, most from Poland and the Soviet Union, had long been commemorated in a beautifully tended war memorial.

The location of the camp at first appeared unremarkable: a desolate, untended field bordered by some battered wooden barracks on one side with a few concrete bunkers at the far end. Yet inside me rose images of living skeletons, acts of persecution and the brutal regimes inflicted daily in the camp. The past seemed present. I was standing where my father's boots had trodden many years before. It chilled me and made the field's emptiness resound.

By extraordinary coincidence, the previous year, while I was researching this book, a museum had opened here, and in a converted barracks there is now a bright, state-of-the-art space with illuminated, life-size images, showcases with found objects from the site, a model of the camp's layout and a library of documents, reports, army communiqués, memoirs and on one shelf, baskets and small figures made from corn stalks by inmates which had been exchanged with the local community for food.

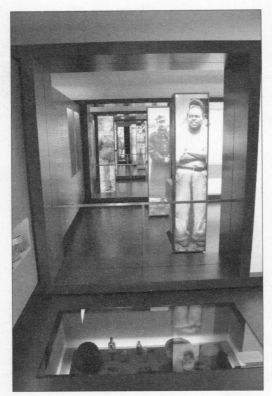

Sandbostel Museum,
near Bremen
(photo © Peter Chappell).

The history of what went on in this abandoned field might have died with those who witnessed it. Instead, in its first year, the creation of the museum has drawn visitors and study groups of students from Russia, Poland, and Germany. Now it is possible to trace their missing grandfathers, and all who come will have resources to raise their own questions, to make connections and to come to their own conclusions. To these resources I have added my father's letters from Sandbostel and the five photographs he took of the concentration camp survivors who, until then, had not been pictured. A small gesture of return.

HOLLY AYLETT, 2015